Donald Monro

An Account of the Diseases which were most frequent in the British

military Hospitals in Germany

From January 1761 to the Return of the Troops to England in March 1763

Donald Monro

An Account of the Diseases which were most frequent in the British military Hospitals in Germany
From January 1761 to the Return of the Troops to England in March 1763

ISBN/EAN: 9783337136185

Printed in Europe, USA, Canada, Australia, Japan

Cover: Foto ©ninafisch / pixelio.de

More available books at **www.hansebooks.com**

AN

ACCOUNT

OF THE

DISEASES

Which were moſt frequent in the

BRITISH MILITARY HOSPITALS
in Germany,

From January 1761 to the Return of the Troops
to England in March 1763.

To which is added,

An ESSAY on the Means of Preſerving the Health
of Soldiers, and conducting Military Hoſpitals.

By DONALD MONRO, M.D.

PHYSICIAN to his MAJESTY's ARMY, and to
ST. GEORGE's Hoſpital.

LONDON:

Printed for A. MILLAR, D. WILSON, and T. DURHAM,
in the Strand, and T. PAYNE, at the Mews Gate.

TO THE

K I N G.

May it pleafe Your MAJESTY,

TO permit me to lay at your Feet the following Sheets, publifhed with a View to be ufeful to thofe, who hereafter may have the Care of the Health of your MAJESTY's Troops.

YOUR

YOUR MAJESTY's particular Inquiries into the State of Your Military Hofpitals, in every Quarter of the World, in the Time of the late glorious and fuccefsful War; Your Concern for every Officer and Soldier who fuffered either by Sicknefs or by Wounds in the Caufe of their King and Country; and Your Solicitude to procure them every poffible Affiftance and Re-lief, cannot fail to excite the higheft Admiration of Your MAJESTY's Goodnefs in the

Breaft

Breaſt of every Subject, and the warmeſt Gratitude in the Heart of every Soldier.

THE Knowledge of theſe Cir-cumſtances induced me to flatter myſelf, that a Work of this Kind would be agreeable to Your MAJESTY; and ſhould this At-tempt towards pointing out the Means of alleviating thoſe Mi-ſeries, which neceſſarily attend a Military Life in the Time of Service, be acceptable, I ſhall obtain the utmoſt of my Wiſhes;

A 3   it

it being the greateſt Ambition
of my Heart ever ſo to act as to
merit Your MAJESTY's Appro-
bation, and to ſubſcribe myſelf,

May it pleaſe Your MAJESTY,

Your MAJESTY's moſt dutiful Subject,

And moſt faithful

and humble Servant,

DONALD MONRO.

THE

PREFACE.

AMONG the numerous Authors
of Obſervations in the Art of
Phyſick, there are but few who have
expreſsly written on the Treatment of
thoſe Diſtempers, moſt generally incident to an Army in the Field : The
following Work, therefore, ſeems to
have a fair Claim to be acceptable to
the Publick, having been compiled
during the Author's Attendance on the

A 4   *Britiſh*

Britiſh Military Hoſpitals in *Germany* in the late War; and in order to render it of ſtill further Uſe, he has occaſionally added, by Way of Note, the Practice of ſome of the moſt eminent Phyſicians in ſimilar Diſeaſes, as well as a few Hiſtories of Caſes which paſſed under his own Care at *St. George's* Hoſpital, *London.*

To avoid the Repetition of the Compoſition of particular Medicines, and the Interruption that would be given by their being inſerted in the Body of the Work, a ſmall Pharmacopœia is added, to which his Practice in the Army Hoſpitals was chiefly confined.

IN

IN a commercial Country like our own, where Numbers of Hands are conftantly wanted for the carrying on our Manufactories, we have a ftrong political Argument to add to that drawn from the Dictates of Humanity, why the Life of every individual fhould be moft carefully attended to.

THE Prefervation of the Lives of Soldiers is then with us a Matter of the higheft Importance, in order to make as low as poffible the Number of Recruits who muft be perpetually drawn off for the Service of War.   The Author has, therefore, in this Treatife, endeavoured to point out the Means moft likely to keep Men healthy when
employed

employed in different Services; and
alfo the Manner in which Military
Hofpitals ought to be fitted up, and
conducted.—As he was never in any
of the warm Climates, nor ever at Sea
along with Troops aboard of Tranfports, whatever is mentioned relative
to fuch Situations, is to be underftood
as taken from printed Accounts of thefe
Subjects, or collected from the Conver-
fation of phyfical Gentlemen, who
were employed on fuch Services during
the two laft Wars.

I T is but Juftice here to obferve,
that the Marquis of *Granby*, Commander in Chief of the *Britifh* Troops
in *Germany*, as well as the Reft of the
General

General Officers employed on the *Ger-man* Service, always paid the greateſt Attention to the Soldiers when ſick in Hoſpitals ; and were particularly ready in giving Orders for all ſuch Things as were neceſſary or proper for them.

JERMYN-STREET,
April 15, 1764.

CONTENTS.

(xiii)

CONTENTS.

Of

Of

xvi C O N T E N T S.

ERRATA CORRIGENDA.

Page 13, line 11, for *Pleuretic*, read *Pleuritic*.
  18,   10, of Notes, for *Acadamy*, read *Academy*.
  28,   22, for *Cinamon*, read *Cinnamon*.
  35,   5, of Notes, for *Calomile*, read *Calomel*.
  51,   12, dele *ufed in this Way*.
  166,   12, of Notes, for *which almoft depend*, read
        which almoft always depend.
  207,   13, of Notes, for *Vena poftarum*, read *Vena por-*
        tarum.
  259,   4, for *appeared*, read *appear:*
  261,   1, of Notes, for *became*, read *become*.
  280,   20, for *Chamamel*, read *Chamæmel*.
  290,   4, for 3^tis 4^tiis, read 3^tiis 4^tis.
  293,   13, for *Mithridatum*, read *Mithridatium*.
  336,   12 & 13, for *bathe themfelves as often*, read
        bathe early in the Morning as often.
  352,   7, for *in Bilanders*, read *and were to go in Bi-*
        landers.
  353,   2, for *the leaft Appearance of the Malignant Fe-*
        ver, read *the Malignant Fever appearing*.

MALIGNANT and PETECHIAL

FEVER.

A Malignant Fever, and Fluxes, began to appear among the Soldiers in Autumn, 1760, while the Allied Army remained encamped about *Warbourg*, from the Beginning of *Auguſt* till the 13th of *December*, when they went into Cantonments. During that Time, there had been a continued Rain for ſome Months, and the Camp and neighbouring Fields, and Villages, were not only filled with the Excrements of ſuch a numerous Army, but likewiſe with infinite Numbers of dead Horſes, and other dead Animals, which had died in doing the neceſſary military Duties, and in bringing Forage, Proviſions, and other

B   Neceſſaries,

Neceffaries, to the Camp: befides this, the Field where there had been an Action on the 31ft of *July*, and where many of the Dead were fcarce covered with Earth, was in the Neighbourhood of the Camp.

Not only the Soldiers, but the Inhabitants of the Country, who were reduced to the greateft Mifery and Want, were infected with the Malignant Fever, and whole Villages almoft laid wafte by it.

Such a Number of Soldiers was fent to *Paderborn* as crowded the Hofpitals there, and increafed the Malignancy of the Diftemper, fo that a great many died.

When I arrived at *Paderborn*, in the Beginning of *January* 1761, the Fever was upon the Decline in the General Hofpitals, though it was ftill rife; but by fending off a Party of Convalefcents to *Herworden*, which thinned the Hofpitals, it became lefs frequent, and but few died. The Guards marched upon the Expedition into *Heffe*, on the eleventh of *February*, which gave us full Room for billetting all our Convalefcents, and thinning the Wards; by which Means the

the Fever almoſt entirely ceaſed in all the Hoſpitals we had before they went away; though there ſtill remained about four hundred ſick.

When the Guards marched out of *Paderborn*, they left the Care of their Sick to us, who belonged to the General Hoſpital: the firſt Regiment of Guards left ſixty ſick; the ſecond, twenty-nine; the third, twenty-eight; and the Granadiers, fifteen, in their regimental Infirmaries; who were moſtly ill of the Malignant Fever: amongſt whom the Infection was ſo very ſtrong, that, although I procured the Sick new airy Houſes for Hoſpitals, which were kept as clean and well-aired as poſſible, and procured clean Bedding, and clean Linen for every Man, and had the Sick laid thin, yet ſeveral died, and it was ſome Time before we got entirely free of the Infection. The firſt and third Regiments ſuffered moſt, owing to all the Sick of each Regiment being put into a particular Hoſpital by themſelves, which kept up the Infection, ſo that they loſt one-third of thoſe left ill of this Fever; and many of the Nurſes, and People who attended them, were ſeized with it. But

not

not being able to procure particular Houſes for the Sick of the *Coldſtream* or Second Regiment, and for the Granadiers, I diſtributed them through the different Hoſpitals we had then in Town, where the Contagion had ceaſed; and by their being thus ſcattered, while they were kept very clean, and at as great a Diſtance as poſſible, from the other Patients in the Wards where they were put, they loſt few in Proportion to the firſt and third Regiments, and the Diſorder did not ſpread.

About the End of *May,* the Weather was very warm at *Oſnabruck*; when this Fever began to make its Appearance in the Corner of a large Ward, which was next to one kept for ſalivating venereal Patients; and only divided from it by means of a few thin Deals. Perceiving a ſtrong Smell in this Place, I ſuſpected that the Fever aroſe from the foul Steams coming from the next Ward, and therefore ordered the ſalivating Ward to be thinned, and removed all the Sick from the Places near that Ward; and ordered thoſe that had catched the Fever to be put into large airy Places; by which means the Infection ſpread no further, and

and only one, out of fix or feven who had got the Fever, died.

At the End of *June*, the Weather was very hot at *Bilifield*, and the Fever began to fhew itfelf by the Hofpital being over-crowded, by a greater Number of Sick being fent from the Army than we had proper Places to put them in ; but it was put a Stop to in a few Days, by the Removal of the Hofpital. Seventy Sick were left behind to the Care of a Mate, moft of them ill of the Fever, of whom twelve died.

In the Beginning of *Auguft*, a few Men were taken ill of the fame Fever at *Munfter*, in one of the Hofpitals which was too much crowded ; but its further Progrefs was ftopped by fending a Number of recovered Men to Billet.

In *November* and *December* 1761, and *January*, *February*, and *March* 1762, we had feveral Men fent from Quarters in the Town of *Bremen* to the Hofpital, fick of the Petechial Fever: they were quartered on the Ground-floors of low damp Houfes, and frefh Meat and Vegetables fo dear that they could

B 3 not

not afford to buy them, but were obliged to live moftly on falt Provifions. I was told like-wife that the fpotted Fever was frequent among the lower Clafs of the Inhabitants. Some few were feized with this Fever in the Hofpi-tal itfelf; yet as the Houfe was not crowded, and we had a Number of fmall airy Wards, the Infection did not fpread; and we had but one or two who died of this Fever during the Winter, in the Hofpital I attended.

In Summer 1762, we had only ten or eleven ill of this Fever in the Hofpital at *Nat-zungen*, and only one died.

When the Troops marched from their Can-tonments, in *December* 1762, towards the Borders of *Holland*, the twentieth and twenty-fifth Regiments of Foot left behind them, at *Ofnabruck*, thirty fick; five of whom had Symp-toms of the Hofpital Fever, though no Pete-chiæ appeared; three recovered, and two died fuddenly, being lodged in large open Wards (the only Places we had to put them in) with the Windows all broke, in very cold frofty Weather.

In

In *January* 1763, we had only three Patients in this Fever, with the Petechiæ upon them, who all recovered. After this we had none taken ill of it at *Ofnabruck,* while I remained there, which was till the twenty-fifth of *March.*

This Malignant Fever begun varioufly in different Subjects; for the moſt part with Cold and Shivering, Pain in the Head, and other Symptoms, commonly defcribed as peculiar to this Fever. In fome, it begun with a fharp Pain of the Side, or other Parts, attended with acute inflammatory Symptoms ; in others, it put on the Appearance of the common, low, or nervous Fever, for a Day or two. Blood drawn in the Beginning from fome Patients did not feem much altered ; from others it threw up a ſtrong inflammatory Buff (*a*) ; but

where

(*a*) Dr. *Huxham,* in his *Treatiſe on the ulcerous ſore Throat,* p. 36, fays, " I have very often met with this buffy or " fizy Appearance of the Blood in the Beginning of Ma‧ " lignant Fevers ; and yet, Blood drawn two or three Days " afterwards, from the fame Perfons, hath been quite loofe, " diffolved, and fanious as it were." And in his *Eſſay on Fe-* *vers,* chap. viii. p. 108. fays, " The firſt Blood frequently

" appears

where the Fever had continued fome time, it was commonly of a loofe Texture, and of a livid Colour; unlefs when the Sick were accidentally feized with pleuretic Stitches, or other Diforders of this kind.

The Reafon of this Difference of Symptoms in the Beginning, and of thefe different Appearances of the Blood, feemed to be, that fuch Patients as laboured under Pleurifies, low or other Fevers, being brought into Hofpitals where the Malignant Fever was frequent, had their original Diforders changed into this Fever by breathing a foul infected Air, and by their Communication with thofe ill of the Fever, and of Fluxes; at other Times, a mere Acrimony of the Blood, fet in Motion by a fupervening Fever, determined the Diforder to be of this kind: and I always obferved, that thofe Men were moft apt to catch this Fever, whofe Con-

" appears floxid; what is drawn twenty-four Hours after, is
" commonly livid, black, and too thin; a third quantity,
" livid, diffolved, and fanious. I have fometimes obferved the
" Crafis of the Blood fo broke as to depofite a black Powder, like
" Soot, at the Bottom, the fuperior Part being either a livid
" Gore, or a dark green, and exceedingly foft Jelly."

ftitutions

ftitutions had been broke down by previous Diforders.

The Fever appeared in different Forms. Some had only a Quicknefs of the Pulfe, attended with a flight Head-ach and Sicknefs, Whitenefs of the Tongue and Thirft, and a Lownefs and Languor; which continued for a Week or more, and then went off, either infenfibly, or with a profufe Sweat, fucceeded by a plentiful Sediment in the Urine. Moft of thofe who fell into profufe kindly-warm Sweats recovered, the Sweat carrying off the Fever. Thefe profufe Sweats continued for twelve or twenty-four Hours, and fometimes for two, three, or four Days. In thofe who had the Fever in this flight Degree, the Petechiæ feldom appeared; and it was only known to be this fort of Fever by the other Symptoms, and the Malignant Fever being frequent at that time in the Hofpitals. Dr. *Pringle* (*b*) very juftly obferves, " That thefe low Degrees of this " Fever are hardly to be characterifed, and are " only to be difcovered, in full Hofpitals, by

(*b*) *Obfervations on the Difeafes of the Army*, part III. chap. vii. fect. 3. third Edition, 1761.

" obferving

" obferving Men languifh ; though the Nature
" of the Illnefs, for which they come in, fhould
" feem to admit of a fpeedier Cure."
For the moft Part the Fever appeared with
more violent Symptoms, the Tongue became
more parched and dry, more or lefs of a Delirium came on, attended with the other
Symptoms commonly defcribed as peculiar to
this Fever.
When the Petechiæ appeared, they came
out on the fourth, fifth, fixth, or feventh
Day; feldom after the eleventh or twelfth (c).
They appeared moftly on the Breaft, Back,

(c) *Ramazini*, in his Treatife *De Conftitutionibus annorum,*
1692, 3. 4, *in Mutinenfi civitate*, Sect. 19. mentions the Petechial Fever which had been frequent the three foregoing
Years; in which the Petechiæ appeared commonly on the
fourth or feventh Days, and almoft all thofe died in whom they
appeared on the firft Day. Thefe Spots came out firft on the
Neck, the Back and Breaft; and it was obferved that none
efcaped unlefs thefe Spots extended themfelves as far as the
Nails of the Toes, vanifhing by Degrees on the upper Parts.
He tells us likewife, that this Fever was attended with an Inflammation of the Throat, which, about the Height of this
Diforder, terminated in a white ulcerous Cruft. This fore
Throat fhould feem to be the fame which we now call *the ma-*
lignant ulcerous fore Throat, which I never once faw while I was
with the Troops in *Germany*.

Arms,

Arms, and Legs, and fometimes, tho' rarely, on the Face. They had exactly the Appearance defcribed by Dr. *Pringle*, either like fmall diftinct Spots of a reddifh Colour, or the Skin looked fometimes as if it had been marbled, or variegated as in the Meafles, but of a Colour more dull and lured. As they began to difappear, they inclined to a dun or brown Colour, and looked like fo many dirty Spots. I never faw them rife above the Skin ; nor did I once fee any miliary Eruptions in this Fever ; which agreed exactly with what Dr. *Pringle* had obferved in the former War, and in the Beginning of this ; however, we ought not to conclude from thence that miliary Eruptions are never obferved in Fevers of this kind; for Dr. *Huxham* (*d*), Dr. *Hafenohrl* (*e*) and Dr. *Lind* (*f*), befides

(*d*) Dr. *Huxham*, in his *Effay on Fevers*, ch. viii. p. 97, tells us, that fometimes, about the eleventh or twelfth Day, on the coming on of profufe Sweats, the Petechiæ difappear, and vaft Quantities of fmall white miliary puftules break out.

(*e*) Dr. *Hafenohrl*, in his Treatife *De Febre Petechiali*, cap. i. p. 12. relates a very particular Cafe, where the Petechiæ appeared on the fourth, and the white miliary Eruptions on the feventeenth Day of the Fever.

(*f*) Dr. *Lind*, in his *fecond Paper on Fevers*, p. 105. mentions

Spots

befides many other good Practitioners, men‐
tion their having feen them.

Many had no Petechiæ through the whole
Courfe of the Diforder; but in all who were
very bad, the Countenance looked bloated, and
the Eyes reddifh and fomewhat inflamed; and
though the Skin was commonly dry, yet the
Perfpiration from the Lungs was ftrong. By
thefe Circumftances one might frequently dif‐
cover that the Patient laboured under the ma‐
lignant Fever, without afking any Queftions.

When Men were taken ill of a Fever, which
we fufpected to be of the malignant kind, our
firft Care was to lay them in airy Places, fepa‐
rate as much as pofiible from the other
Men, and to keep them extremely clean;
and they were put on low Diet, and allowed
as much Barley or Rice-water as they chofe to
drink, which was commonly ordered to be aci‐
dulated with the *Spiritus Vitrioli.*

Spots which rife above the Surface of the Skin, and are of the
miliary kind, as common in contagious Fevers, as he obferved
among the *French* Prifoners in *Winchefter* Caftle, in the Be‐
ginning of the Year 1761.

For

Fcr the firft two or three Days we could feldom diftinguifh, with Certainty, that the Fever was of the malignant kind, though we had often Reafon to fufpect it. The Pain of the Head, the Fulnefs and Quicknefs of the Pulfe, and other Symptoms, led us commonly to take away more or lefs Blood, which the Patient bore eafily, and for the moft part it gave Relief(*g*). We feldom repeated this Evacuation where we fufpected the Fever to be of the malignant kind, unlefs a pleuretic Stitch, an acute Pain of the Bowels, or fome other accidental Symptom, required it ; cr the Patient was ftrong, and there were evident Symptoms of Fullnefs immediately before we

(*g*) Dr. *Huxham*, tho' he fays " yet Bleeding to fome Degree " is moft commonly requifite, nay neceffary, in the ftrong and " plethoric ;" yet he afterwards makes the following Remark : " Befides, the Pulfe in thefe Cafes finks oftentimes furprifingly " after a fecond Bleeding, nay fometimes after the firft, and " that even where I thought I had fufficient Indications from " the Pulfe to draw Blood a fecond time." See his *Effay on Fevers*, chap. viii. And Dr. *Pringle* obferves, that in the fecond Stage of the Diforder large Bleedings have generally proved fatal, by finking the Pulfe, and bringing on a Delirium. *Obfervations on the Difeafes of the Army*, part III. chap. vii. fect. V.

intended

intended giving the Bark, as fhall be mentioned afterwards; for under other Circumftances,
if the Blooding was repeated, and other Evacuations ufed freely, I always obferved that it
did Harm, and was apt to fink the Patient too
much; as Dr. *Huxham*, Dr. *Pringle*, and
other good Practitioners, have remarked.

After Bleeding, if the Patient was coftive, or complained of Gripes, he had a Dofe
of Rhubarb, or Salts, or a laxative Clyfter; but where there was much Sicknefs
of the Stomach, we gave a gentle Emetic (*b*)
in the Evening, and the Purge next Morning.

And

(*b*) Dr. *Pringle* advifes giving a Vomit, by way of Prevention, on the firft Appearance of the Symptoms, and at Night to
force a Sweat, by giving a Drachm of Theriac with ten Grains
Sal volat. Corn. cervi, and fome Draughts of Vinegar-whey,
and to repeat the fame the following Night; and fays, he has
often feen thofe Symptoms removed which he apprehended to
be Forerunners of this Fever received by Contagion ; but previous to Vomits, or Sweats, if the Perfon be plethoric, it will
be neceffary to take away fome Blood. *Obferv.* part III. ch. vii.
fect. 5. Dr. *Lind*, in his *fecond Paper on Fevers*, p. 66. fays;
" To all who are fuppofed to be infected by Fevers, during
" this Stage of Rigours, a gentle Vomit is immediately
" to be exhibited before the Fever be formed, and before the
" Fulnefs or Hardnefs of the Pulfe renders its Operation dan-
" gerous.

And if in the Courſe of the Diſorder the Sickneſs and Nauſea returned, attended with Griping and Coſtiveneſs, or very fetid looſe Stools, theſe Medicines were repeated, and a gentle Opiate given in the Evening after their Operation.

After Evacuations, if the Pulſe kept up, we commonly gave nothing but the ſaline Draughts, with the *Pulvis contrayervæ*, or ſome temperate Medicine, for the firſt Day or two. As ſoon as we could diſtinguiſh the Fever to be of the malignant kind, and that the Pulſe rather ſunk, we joined ſome of the Cordials to the ſaline Medicines, and allowed the Patient

" gerous. If the Vomit be delayed too long, and eſpecially if
" Bleeding muſt precede it, the moſt certain and favoura-
" ble Opportunity of procuring Safety for the Patient is
" paſt. —— That he has found it equally ſerviceable in
" preventing Relapſes, when it is given at the Return of the
" Shiverings." A looſe Stool, or two, ſhould be procured
by the Emetic or Clyſters, and he adviſes Sweating immediately after, in the manner recommended by Dr *Pringle*. At
other times " he gave five Grains of Camphire every four
" Hours, with large Draughts of Vinegar-whey. Eight
" Perſons in ten, he ſays, got quite well by this Treatment."

I have never had ſufficient Opportunities of trying this
Method of Prevention, to determine any thing certain about
it ; but it may be worth while to practiſe it.

more

more or lefs Wine, according to the Degree
of the Fever.   Dr. *De Haen* has found Fault
with Dr. *Pringle* and Dr. *Huxham*, for admi-
niftering cordial Medicines and Wine in the
low State of this Fever; but nothing anfwered
fo well with us as thefe Remedies under fuch
Circumftances ; and I have frequently feen
every Symptom changed for the better by their
Ufe ; and even when I gave the Bark, in the
Manner recommended by *De Haen*, I often
found it neceflary to join the free Ufe of Wine(*i*),
Cordials

(*i*) *Petrus a Caftro*, in his Account of a Petechial Fever,
which was frequent at *Verona*, tells us, that the Sick had a
great Thirft, and an Averfion to Meat, but all of them had
the ftrongeft Defire for Wine, and were perpetually afking for
it, even thofe who at other Times ufed to be very temperate ;
and that this proceeded from an Inftinct of Nature, which wanted
fomething to fupport the Strength. *De Feb. Malig.* fect. iii. chap.
26. Dr. *Huxham*, in his *Effay on Fevers*, has the following very
judicious Remark on the Ufe of Wine : " In this View, and in
" thofe above-mentioned, I cannot but recommend a generous red
" Wine as a moft noble, natural fub-aftringent Cordial, and per-
" haps Art can fcarce fupply a better.   Of this I am confident,
" that fometimes at the State, and more frequently in the De-
" cline of putrid Malignant Fevers, it is of the higheft Service,
" efpecially when acidulated with Juice of *Seville* Orange or
" Lemon.   It may be alfo impregnated with fome Aromatics,
" as Cinamon, *Seville* Orange Rhind, red Rofes, or the like, as
                                                  . " may

Cordials and Blisters (*k*), in order to support the Patient's Strength.

" may be indicated, and a few Drops of *Elix. Vitrioli* may be
" added. Rhenish and French White Wines, diluted, make a
" most salutary Drink in several Kinds of Fevers, and generous
" Cyder is little inferior to either. The *Afiatics*, and other
" Nations, where pestilential Disorders are much more rife
" than with us, lay more Stress on the Juice of Lemons in
" these Fevers than on the most celebrated *Alexipharmac.*" Chap.
viii. second Edit. p. 123, 4.

Acid and acefcent Liquors have very justly been recommended and used by most late Practitioners, in this as well as
in other malignant Difeases. Vinegar-whey, Barley-water acidulated with Lemon-juice, and such other Liquors, make good
Drinks for the Sick; but we were obliged, for the most part,
to use the vitriolic Acid for acidulating the Patient's Drink,
as it was the easiest procured and carried about with the Flying
Hospital.

(*k*) If the preventive Method does not succeed, Dr. *Lind*
advifes to have recourfe to Blisters ; and says, that sixteen out
of twenty will next Morning be free of the Fever. But adds,
this is said, provided the Source of their Infection be not fo
highly poisonous as it was in the Garland Ship, or in other
such violent Contagions. Dr. *Pringle* mentions his having applied Blisters early, but without relieving the Head, or preventing any of the usual Symptoms. I have often ordered
Blisters pretty early in the Diforder; and though I have frequently found them of use in keeping up the Pulfe, and relieving the Head, and other Symptoms, yet I never faw them
have such an immediate Effect as Dr. *Lind* mentions.

C   After

After reading the Treatifes of Dr. *De Haen* and Dr. *Hafenohrl,* on this Fever, I refolved on giving the Bark (*l*) in large Quantities, and found it to anfwer the Recommendations given by thefe Gentlemen ; and fhall relate here two or three Cafes, out of above a hundred and fifty, in which I gave it.

I. *Robert Wilfon,* of the Second Regiment of Foot Guards, on the 19th of *February* 1761, was feized with a Shivering and Coldnefs, fuc-

(*l*) It is long fince the *Peruvian* Bark has been ufed by Practitioners in Malignant Diforders, though I do not know that any body gave it in this Fever to the Amount of an Ounce per Day, before Dr. *Haen* and Dr. *Hafenohrl.* Dr. *Ramazini* mentions its having been tried in the Petechial Fever, in the Years 1692, 3, 4. And in a Treatife on the Plague in the *Ucrane,* publifhed at *Petersburgh,* in the Year 1750, we are told, that in the *French* Tranflation of the Philofophical Tranfactions for the Year 1732, there is a Note to p. 264, telling, that Mr. *Amyand* informed the Acadamy of Surgery at *Paris,* that Mr. *Rufhworth,* Surgeon, had wrote to Sir *Hans Sloane,* on the 23d of *May* 1723, that when he was Surgeon to a Ship, in the Year 1694, he had cured fome Men ill of the Malignant Fever, attended with peftilential Buboes, by means of the *Peruvian* Bark. Dr. *Huxham* has recommended a Tincture of the Bark ; and Dr. *Pringle,* a ftrong Decoction of it, with fome of the Tincture, in thefe Malignant Fevers.

ceeded

ceeded with Heat, Thirst, a short dry Cough, Difficulty of Breathing, Head-ach, and slight Stitches in his Breast; some Blood was taken away, which was fizy, and he was ordered two Ounces of the *Sperma Ceti* Mixture, with the *spiritus mindereri*, every two or three Hours. He continued without any manifest Alteration in the Symptoms, till the 21st, when a Number of dun Petechiæ appeared all over his Body, particularly on his Breast. The Stitches and Cough were then much easier, and he had his Medicines as before. On the 22d, he was seized with a Delirium, and was somewhat comatose; when he was ordered a Drachm of the Bark every six Hours. The 23d, the comatose Symptoms had increased, and he had slight Twitchings of the Tendons, a dry brown-coloured Tongue, and a Faultering in his Speech. The Bark was continued, with the Addition of two Spoonfuls of Mountain Wine every two Hours. On the 24th, he had several loose Stools. The 25th, he was still loose, and went on as before, with the Addition of six Grains of the *Pilulæ fapona-*

C 2   *cœ*

cæ in the Evening. The 26th, the Petechiæ were not fo apparent as before, but he had ftill the nervous Symptoms, and his Breathing grew more difficult; and therefore a Blifter was applied between his Shoulders, and his Medicines continued; as they were likewife on the 27th, without any Alteration in the Symptoms. On the 28th, his Tongue became moifter, and the Pulfe, which had been low and quick the four preceding Days, became fuller and flower. On the 29th, he was much more fenfible, his Tongue more moift, and the Twitchings of the Tendons much lefs; and in the Evening he fell into a profufe Sweat, which lafted all the 30th. On the 1ft of *March,* his feverifh Symptoms were much abated, his Pulfe was calmer, his Skin moift, his Drought lefs, and his Urine dropt a plentiful Sediment. On the 2d, his Fever was almoft entirely gone, but he had ftill a Cough, and fpit up a vifcid Matter. He was ordered to go on as before, with the Addition of two Spoonfuls of the *Sperma Ceti* Mixture, and the *Spiritus Mindereri,* when

his

his Cough was troublefome. He followed this Courfe till the 7th, when, his Cough
and Fever being gone, he was ordered a
Dofe of Tincture of Rhubarb ; after which he
recruited his Strength daily, without the Affiftance of any more Medicines.

II. On the 5th of *March* 1761, *Thomas Stagg*,
of the Second Regiment of Foot Guards,
was feized with the fame Symptoms as *Robert
Wilfon* had been in the Beginning of his Fever,
but in a more violent Degree. He was blooded
to about twelve Ounces, and was ordered a faline
Draught every fix Hours. On the 6th, the
Blood, which had been drawn the Day before,
had thrown up a flight Buff ; it appeared to
contain but a fmall Proportion of Serum, and
the Craffamentum was of a loofe Texture.
The feverifh Symptoms had increafed, with
the Addition of a Delirium : pergat. On the
7th, the Delirium was grown more violent, fo
that he could fcarce be kept in Bed; his Breathing was difficult, his Eyes red and florid : A
Blifter was applied to his Back, and the faline
Mixture continued. On the 8th, there was
no Alteration in the Courfe of that Day ; but

being

being lower towards Night, Blifters were applied to his Legs, and he was ordered to have a
Pint of Wine allowed him in twenty-four
Hours. On the 9th, the Petechiæ appeared
over his whole Body, of a broad dunnifh kind;
his Breathing became eafier, and his Pulfe
ftronger, though the Delirium was ftill as
bad as before : He was ordered a Drachm of
the Bark every fourth Hour in a faline Draught.
On the 10th, the Bark gave him feveral loofe
Stools, but the Petechiæ were of a more florid
Colour; the Delirium was lefs, and his Tongue
moift, and therefore he was ordered to continue the fame Medicines as the Day before,
with the Addition of ten Grains of the *Pilulæ
faponaceæ* in the Evening. The 11th Day,
he fell into a fine breathing Sweat, his Pulfe
became fuller and flower, and the Delirium
abated : p. The 12th, his Pulfe was regular,
and the Delirium gone, and he was much
inclined to fleep. The 13th, after a calm
Sleep, which had lafted twelve or fourteen
Hours, he became quite free of Fever. After this he continued the Ufe of his Medicines

cines for fome Days, and recovered his Health
and Strength daily.

III. On the 23d of *May* 1761, *Lionel Thomp-
fon*, of the Firſt Regiment of Foot Guards,
was feized with all the Symptoms of a Peripneumony, attended with a high Fever, for
which he was ordered to be blooded. After
lofing eight Ounces of Blood, he fell into a
fainting Fit ; on recovering out of which, his
Breathing being ſtill much affected, he had a
Mixture made of four Ounces of the *Lac Ammoniacum*, and one of the *ſpiritus mindereri*,
of which he was defired to take two Spoonfuls
every four Hours. The 24th, the Symptoms
the fame : He complained of having had no
Stool for fome Days, and took half an Ounce
of the *fal catharticum amarum*, which gave
him two loofe Stools. On the 25th, his Pulfe
was fmall and quick, his Breathing difficult; he
was low, and had a ſlight Delirium : A large
Blifter was applied between his Shoulders, and
the Medicines continued. On the 26th, in
the Morning, the Petechiæ appeared, and
his Breathing was freer : He was ordered a
Drachm of the Bark, in a faline Draught, every

C 4   four

four Hours. The 27th, the Pulfe better: p. The 28th, was more fenfible, and had a kindly warm Moifture all over the Skin. The 29th, the Fever was much abated, and his Tongue, which was before parched and dry, became moift and white: He continued the Ufe of the Cortex for three Days more, which removed the Fever; and being coftive, he took a Dofe of the Tincture of Rhubarb. After this he ufed the Bark for a few Days longer, and got perfectly well.

After giving the Bark (*m*) with Succefs, in the two firft of the Cafes mentioned, and to two

young

(*m*) The *Peruvian* Bark has not only been found ufeful in this Malignant Fever, but has likewife been recommended in the Plague. See *Morton Oper. Append. fecund. Exercitat. Hift. Febr. Ann.* 1658, *ad. an.* 1691. *complexa.* In the Small Pox, fee *Medical Effays,* vol. V. art. *x.* and has been found ferviceable in the putrid Diforders of the *Weft-Indies,* as taken Notice of by Dr. *Hillary;* and in the malignant ulcerous fore Throat in this Country, as Dr. *Wall* and others have obferved. And in thirty-five Cafes of the malignant ulcerous fore Throat, in which I gave it, joined with Cordials, and the Ufe of Acids, I did not lofe one Patient. Nine of them were ftrong People, and had plethoric Symptoms, and were blooded in the Begin-ning; and feven of them were coftive, and took a Dofe of gen-

tle

young Gentlemen, Mates of the Hofpital, who had caught the Fever from their Attendance on the Sick, I gave it to above a hundred and fifty at *Paderborn,* and elfewhere, during my Attendance in the Military Hofpitals in *Germany*; and although it did not anfwer in every Cafe, yet it was found to have a better Effeçt than any other Remedy that was tried. We joined different Medicines with it, according to the State of the Patient   We gave the *Confeçtio cardiaca, Rad. ferpent. Virg.* and other cordial Medicines, and Wine, when the Pulfe was low; *Oxymel fcilliticum,* and other Peçtorals, when

tle laxative Phyfic before taking the Bark.   The reft had no Symptoms which feemed to require thefe Evacuations.   However, it ought to be obferved, that this is a Diforder of the malignant kind ; and that although fome well-timed gentle Evacuations may be ferviceable in the Beginning, before giving the Bark ; yet too free, or even gentle Evacuations, injudicioufly made, will fink the Patient, and infallibly do Mifchief.

The free Ufe of the Bark has long been found ferviceable in Mortifications and foul Sores, where the Juices tend too much to the Putrefcent ; and has been ftrongly recommended by Mr. *Ranby,* Serjeant Surgeon to his Majefty, in the Cure of Gunfhot Wounds.   See his *Treatife on Gunfhot Wounds.*

the

the Breathing was difficult; Opiates, where the
Patient was inclined to be too loofe; the *fpiritus mindereri*, and other Diaphoretics, when
we wanted to promote a free Perfpiration; and
we applied Blifters as Occafion required.

When the Patient was ftrong, the Pulfe
quick and full, the Eyes looked red, and the
Breathing was difficult, after the Petechiæ appeared; I took away more or lefs Blood before
giving the Bark. Moft Practitioners of late
Years have been againft Bleeding in this Stage
of the Diforder; but trufting to the Affurances
given by Dr. *Hafenobrl* of its being fafe, nay of
Advantage to bleed at this Time, if the Symptoms required it, I ventured upon it, and found
it to be of the greateft Service, in many Cafes,
in the Hofpitals at *Paderborn* and elfewhere;
and particularly in two Cafes at *Bremen*, and
one at *Ofnabruck*, where it gave immediate Relief, and feemed to fhorten the Difeafe much.
One of the Patients at *Bremen, Robert Ellis*,
belonged to an Independant Company; the other,
Francis Hamftan, of the 24th Regiment, had formerly had his Skull fractured, and took the Fever,
while he was in the Hofpital, for violent Head-
achs,

achs, which he had been fubject to, at times, ever after his Skull had been fractured. The Cafe at *Ofnabruck* was a Nurfe of the Hofpital, whofe Name was —— *Andrews,* a Woman about twenty-five Years of Age, who, after attending a Dragoon in the Small Pox, and fuckling at the fame time her own Child, then in the fame Diforder, was, on the 18th of *January* 1763, attacked with a Fever. I faw her for the firft time on the 20th, and found her Pulfe quick, full, and ftrong. She complained of a violent Head-ach ; for which fhe was blooded, and took the faline Mixture, with Nitre and Contrayerva. Next Day, the 21ft, her Blood appeared very fizy, and fhe complained of having been coftive for fome Days. We gave her immediately an Ounce of the *fal catharticum amarum,* which operated well. She continued much in the fame Way the 22d, and had fome loofe Stools that Day. Being ftill inclined to be loofe the 23d, inftead of her former Medicines, fhe was ordered the *fpiritus mindereri* Mixture, with Mithridate. This checked the Purging, but did not ftop it entirely. The Fever

ver went on, without any remarkable Change, till the 27th; at which time the Petechiæ appeared all over her Body, attended with a Redness of the Eyes, and a violent Oppreſſion and Pain of her Head, and a quick Pulſe. I ordered ſix Ounces of Blood to be taken away immediately, and a large Bliſter to be applied to her Back, and, at the ſame time, ordered her a cordial Mixture, with half an Ounce of the Extract of the Bark in it, to be taken every twenty-four Hours. The 28th, her Pulſe was not ſo hard, her Head was much eaſier, the Redneſs of her Eyes was much leſs, and the Petechiæ had begun to die away. The Blood which was taken away the Day before, had a thin Buff at the Top, but the *Craſſamentum* underneath was of a dark Colour, and of a looſe Texture: p. On the 29th, ſhe told me that ſhe had had two or three looſe Stools, and ſhe was lower than the Day before; and therefore a Drachm of Mithridate, and two Drachms of the Tincture of Cinamon, were added to her cordial Mixture, with the Cortex; and ſhe was allowed half a Pint of Red Wine, mulled with

Cinamon,

Cinamon, *per* Day.   30th, Her Tongue rather moifter than the Day before ; and fhe not fo low, but fhe was ftill inclined to be loofe; and therefore was ordered the anodyne Draught at Nights, and to continue the other Medicines.   31ft, She was ftill inclined to be loofe; but her Pulfe kept up, her Tongue was moifter, and fhe foundherfelf pretty eafy : p. *Feb.* 1ft, Her Pulfe pretty ftrong, and fhe found herfélf much cooler, and freer from the Fever, and complained of a Dullnefs of Hearing.   On the 2d, in the Morning, fhe felt a warm Moifture all over her Skin, which, about Noon, broke out into a profufe Sweat, and continued till the 4th ; when it went off, and her Urine let fall a copious whitifh Sediment.   She had then little or no Fever.   The Dullnefs of Hearing ftill continued, though it was much lefs than before.   After this the Deafnefs went gradually away.   She continued the Ufe of the cordial Mixture, with the Cortex, till the 12th, and recovered Strength daily.   After this, fhe had no other Medicine, except two Dofes of the Tincture of Rhubarb, and

and was foon in good Health, and able to dif-charge her Duty as a Nurfe.

However, it ought to be obferved, that we muft not bleed fo freely, in this or any other Stage of the Malignant Fever, as in acute inflam-matory Diforders, otherwife we fhall fink the Pa-tient, and hurry him to his Grave; and that Bleeding can only take place with Safety and Advantage, under the Circumftances above-mentioned, immediately before giving the Bark freely; or where fome accidental fharp Pain in the Breaft, or Bowels, or fome other violent Symptom, may require it. They err equally, who recommend Bleeding freely in this Fever, with thofe who entirely forbid its Ufe.

Although we found the Bark to be in general the beft Remedy in this malignant Petechial Fever, yet it did not anfwer in every Cafe; for in fome we found other Remedies had a better Effect: And therefore, when we obferved that, notwithftanding the Ufe of the Bark, the Pa-tient funk, and the Symptoms grew worfe, we did not perfift obftinately in its Ufe, but tried the Effect of other Medicines.

Towards

Towards the End of *May* 1761, two Soldiers in the Hofpital, at *Ofnabruck*, were taken ill of this Fever; who, after ufing the Bark freely, and being allowed a Pint of Red Wine *per* Day, for fome Days together, began to fink, and had a Delirium and other bad Symptoms haftening on: upon which I laid afide the Ufe of the Bark, and ordered each of them a Blifter to the Back, and to take a cordial Draught, with fifteen Grains of Mufk in it, every four Hours; and to have their Wine mulled with Cinamon; and although at that Time they were both fo low that I fcarce imagined they would live twenty-four Hours, yet next Day I found them greatly mended; and they had a kindly warm Moifture all over their Skin, and the Pulfe had rofe confiderably in both. By the Continuance of the fame Medicine the feverifh Symptoms gradually abated, and they both got well.

About the fame time, having given the Bark freely for fome Days, and applied a Blifter, to another Patient, after the Petech'æ had appeared, I found him one Morring fo low that his

Pulfe

Pulfe could fcarce be felt. He could not fpeak; he had a Delirium, and rather a Tremor than a *fubfultus tendinum*, and he had all the Appearance of a dying Man. However, as he ftill fwallowed whatever was put in his Mouth, I changed the Bark Mixture for Draughts, which contained a Scruple of the *confeɛtio cardiaca*, and feven Grains of the *fal vol. corn. cerv.* (*n*) each,

(*n*) Dr. *Huxham*, in his *Treatife cn the ulcerous fore Throat*, p. 54, &c. condemns the Ufe of the volatile alcaline Salts, in Fevers of the putrid, peftilential, or petechial kind, as being apt to heat tco much, and to haften the Diffolution and confequent Putrefaɛtion of the Blood. However, I cannot help thinking that they are the beft Remedies we can ufe on fome particular Occafions, even in this Fever; for we have no Remedy which gives fuch a fudden and brifk *Stimulus* to the Fibres as they do. And I have known many Cafes of Patients who were extremely low, and whofe Pulfe was fcarce to be felt, and others who were apt to fall into fainting Fits, who have been preferved by large and repeated Dofes of thefe Salts, and the free Ufe of Wine, and acefcent Liquors, to correɛt their alcaline Acrimony in the Blood. Though as foon as fuch Patients had recovered from this low State, I laid thefe Medicines afide; becaufe I cannot help agreeing with the Doɛtor in the Belief, that their continued Ufe will produce the Effeɛts he mentions. For although it be true, that thefe Salts, when mixed with putrefcent Liquors, or with dead animal Subftances, refift Putrefaction,

each, and ordered one to be given immediately, and afterwards to be repeated every four Hours ; and, in the Intervals, to give him frequently a Tea-cup full of Red Wine, mulled with Cinnamon ; and to apply two large Blifters to his Legs. Next Day, his Pulfe had rofe ; and by the Continuance of the fame Remedies it became gradually fuller and ftronger, and the third Day after he recovered his Voice ; and a warm kindly Moif-ture which ended in a profufe Sweat coming on, the feverifh Symptoms went off foon after, and he recovered his Health.

At *Bremen* there were two Men, one in *Ja-nuary*, and the other in *February* 1762, on whom the Cortex had but little Effect, who recovered by the free Ufe of Mixtures, with the *confectio cardiaca* and *rad. ferpentariæ*, and

tion, and, like ardent Spirits and Vinegar (the other Products of Fermentation) check and put a Stop to that very Procefs which produced them : Yet it is alfo true, that, when mixed with the Blood of living Animals, they ftimulate the Veffels, and increafe the Heat and *Momentum* of the Blood, and diffolve it ; and therefore I cannot but difapprove the continuing their Ufe longer than is immediately neceffary.

D   of

of Wine, with the Application of large Blifters. Several Cafes of this kind occurred in
the Hofpitals, where the Bark did not anfwer.

There is one thing to be obferved with re-
fpect to Malignant Fevers, which is, that if
ever they appear in large crowded Hofpitals,
unlefs we can thin the Wards, and procure
a free Circulation of Air, and keep the Hofpital and Sick extremely clean, the Fevers will
continue to fpread, and great Numbers will die;
and even the moft efficacious Remedies will
have little or no Effect.   And that when once
the Infection is grown ftrong, it requires the
greateft Care, and fome Time, before it can be
entirely got the better of.   And that if a great
number of Men, ill of this Fever, be kept in
the fame Ward, they will help to keep up the
Infection; and therefore it is always proper,
when it can poffibly be done, to lay but a few
of them in one Ward; not above one-third of
the Number generally admitted.

Many of the Patients, towards the Height
of this Fever, fooner or later, had a Purging,
which feldom proved critical; and fome were

feized

feized with the Flux. A gentle *diarrhœa*, fuch as did not fink the Patient, was commonly of Service ; but when violent, or a Dyfentery came on, the Cafe was always dangerous; for whatever ftopped the Flux increafed the Fever ; and, if the Purging or Flux continued, it funk the Patient. Such Fluxes we treated in the Manner to be mentioned afterwards, when we come to the Hiftory of the Dyfentery.

In this Fever, it was common for Patients to vomit Worms (*n*), or to pafs them by Stool, or, what was more frequent, to have them come up into their Throat and Mouth, or fometimes into their Noftrils, while they were afleep in Bed, and to pull them out with their Fingers. The fame Thing happened to moft of the *Britifh* Soldiers, brought to the Hofpitals for other feverifh Diforders as well as this. Dr. *Pringle* (*o*),

(*n*) Some Men paffed only one Worm ; others, two or three ; fome, fix or feven ; and one Man, of the Guards, in *January* 1763, after paffing three by Stools in the Courfe of a Fever of this Kind, difcharged fourteen more upon taking a Dofe of Rhubarb and Calomile after the Fever was over.

(*o*) *Obfervations on the Difeafes of the Army,* part iii. chap. iv. Note to p. 213. third Edition.

when

when he mentions Worms being obferved in this Fever, feems to embrace *Lancifius*'s Opinion; and believes that thefe Worms are not the Caufe of the Fever; but being lodged in the Inteftines, before the Fever comes on, they are annoyed by the Increafe of the Heat, and the Corruption of the Humours, in the Cavity of the Inteftines of Perfons labouring under Fevers, efpecially of the putrid Kind; and fo they begin to move and ftruggle to get out. This feemed evidently to be the Cafe with many of the Patients we had; though in fome the Worms feemed to have given Rife to the Fever, which the bad State of the Patient's Humours, or the infected Air of Hofpitals, determined to be of this Kind. In many, the Fever leffened, or went off entirely, foon after; and they were no more affected with Symptoms of Worms. But fome notwithftanding were fubject to frequent Sicknefs, Pain of the Stomach, and Uneafinefs in the Bowels, and difcharged fome Worms from Time to Time. Others had frequent Relapfes into Fevers, which feemed to be owing to the Irritation of thefe Infects.

It

It is no Wonder that Worms of the round Kind fhould be produ&ive of troublefome Symptoms, and occafion thefe Relapfes; fince we know that they have fometimes perforated the Inteftines, and been found in the Cavity of the Abdomen (*p*).

As foon as we obferved a Patient to be troubled with Worms, if his prefent Situation did not prevent it, we gave twenty-five or thirty Grains of Rhubarb, with five or fix Grains of Calomel; and if there was much Sicknefs, we likewife gave an Emetic; which, in more than one Cafe, brought up two or three Worms of the round Kind, and gave great Relief. But where the Fever was violent, we were obliged to negle& this Symptom of Worms for the prefent; and when the Fever was over, if there ftill

(*p*) See *Hoffman's* Works, vol. III. chap. x. *River. Obferv. commun.* Obf. 13. *of Obfervations found in a Library. Bonetus's Sepulchret. anatom.* tom. II. *Gualther van Doeveren's Inaugural Differtation de Vermibus inteftinalibus*, publifhed at *Leyden*, 1753; and *Lancifi's* Works; for Cafes where the internal Coats of the Stomach, and Inteftines, have been eroded, and all the Coats perforated by Worms of the round Kind.

remained

remained any Symptoms of Worms, we gave
the purgative Medicine once or oftener, and in
the Intervals gave the *pulvis ſtanni*, or an Infuſion
of Camomile Flowers ; and in ſome Caſes, oily
Medicines.   By theſe Means moſt of the Pati-
tients got well and recovered their Health, and
ſeemed to be freed, at leaſt for the preſent, from
theſe troubleſome Inſects ; though a few con-
nued to complain of Sickneſs, and other Symptoms of Worms, for ſome Time afterwards.

What was the Cauſe of the Army's being ſo
much troubled with Worms of the round Kind,
is not eaſy to aſcertain ; unleſs it was owing to
the great Quantity of crude Vegetables, and
Fruits, which the Soldiers eat in the Courſe of
the Summer and Autumn, and to the bad Water
they were often obliged to drink.

In the Malignant Fever at *Paderborn*, many
complained of a Dyſuria, and ſome of a Suppreſ-
ſion of Urine, eſpecially towards the Decline
of the Fever ; and others, of a Scalding and
Pain in making Water, though they had no venereal Complaint.   Theſe Symptoms appeared
in other Places, but not near ſo frequently as at
Paderborn.

Paderborn. Decoctions of Gum Arabic, with fome of the *fpiritus nitri dulcis*, and oily Mixtures, and Opiates, commonly gave immediate Relief, and foon removed this Complaint.

One of the firft falutary Symptoms which moft generally appeared in thofe who recovered, was a Dullnefs of Hearing, or Deafnefs *(q)*; which came on about the Height of the Fever, and continued a longer or fhorter Time, generally till the Fever was entirely gone ; and fometimes for a confiderable Time afterwards. For the

(q) *Riverius* tells us, that, according to *Hippocrates*'s Doctrine, Deafnefs is a very dangerous Symptom in the Beginning of acute Diforders, though it be a good Omen, and portends Health, when it does not appear till the Height of Fevers, efpecially thofe of a malignant Kind ; and adds, that he himfelf has a thoufand Times obferved, that thofe labouring under this Fever have recovered, when this Symptom of Deafnefs came on at the Height (*in ftatu*) though the other Symptoms threatened much Danger. *Prax. Medic.* lib. XVII. fect. iii. cap. i. p. 451.

This Symptom of Deafnefs occurs in other Fevers as well as in this, and often proves a good Symptom in them likewife, as I have frequently obferved. Two remarkable Examples of which I had under my Care in St. *George*'s Hofpital, in the Year 1759. On the 17th of *January* 1759, *James Donaldfon*, a young Man of nineteen Years of Age, was admitted into the Hofpital for a Fever,

the moft Part we did nothing for this Complaint, and it went off as the Patient recovered his Strength.   When it continued long,
Blifters applied behind the Ears, or on the
Neck, and wafhing the *meatus auditorius* with
the emollient Decoction, in which a fmall Quantity of Soap was diffolved, proved of Service.

Swellings of the parotid Glands appeared in
many Subjects, towards the Decline of the Fever, which came to Suppuration, and proved
critical.   In two only, out of thofe I attended
while in *Germany*, they came on early in the Fe-

ver, attended with a Stupor and a Delirium, a parched dry
Tongue, and other Symptoms of a Fever of the inflammatory
Kind, for which he had been blooded, and ufed other Evacuations.   On the 19th, after the Application of a Blifter, he was
feized with almoft an entire Deafnefs ; after which, all his other
Symptoms became milder, and he mended daily, and was entirely free from the Fever by the 30th.   On the 10th of *April*
1759, a Youth, *John Young*, fifteen Years of Age, was admitted
into the fame Hofpital for a Fever, which had already continued fourteen Days.   His Speech was affected, and he had entirely loft the Ufe of his Limbs, was delirious, and had other
bad Symptoms. On the 12th, his Hearing became exceedingly
dull, and he recovered daily afterwards, and was difcharged,
cured, the 2d of *May*, having recovered the Ufe of his Legs as
well as got free of the Fever.

ver, but did not fuppurate. Both Patients died ; all the reft recovered, except one old Man, an Invalid at *Bremen* ; who, after having one Swelling appear on the right Side, which came to Suppuration, and feemed critical, relapfed into the Fever; and another formed on the other Side, which came likewife to Suppuration, and the Fever ceafed, after having reduced him very low ; but the great Difcharge from the Sores wafted him gradually, and he died hectic in about a Month after the Fever had left him (*r*).

(*r*) But although thefe parotid Swellings were in general fo favourable with us, we are not to imagine that this will always be the Cafe : for *Riverius*, though he fpeaks of thefe Swellings proving for the moft part critical ; yet he tells us, that, in the Year 1623, this Fever was epidemic at *Montpelier*, and that almoft one half of the Sick died ; and particularly, that moft of thofe who had Swellings of the parotid Glands appearing about the 9th or 11th Day, were carried off within two Days of their Appearance. Having attended feveral who died from the Swellings not coming to Suppuration, he began to confider in his own Mind, what might be the Caufe of their Death, and concluded, that it was owing to there being a greater Quantity of morbid Matter in the Blood than the Part was able to contain, and that Evacuations by blooding and purging were the only Remedies which were likely to give Relief ; and therefore, in the firft Cafe of this Kind, in which he was afterwards confulted, he or-

dered

As foon as thefe Swellings of the parotid Glands appeared, we endeavoured to bring them forward to Suppuration, by the Application of emollient Cataplafms, or of gummous Plaifters; and had them opened as foon as a Fluctuation of Matter was to be felt, and afterwards treated them as common Abfceffes. *Riverius* (*s*) very juftly obferves, that when fuch Tumours encreafe in fuch a Manner as to endanger Suffocation, they ought to be opened before they come to Maturation ; and Dr. *Pringle* (*t*) defires us not to wait for a Fluctuation of Matter, but to open the Abfcefs as foon as it can be fuppofed to have formed.

dered three Ounces of Blood to be taken away, notwithftanding the Patient was fo low that the Surgeon was afraid he would have died in the Operation : The Pulfe rofe on bleeding, and he ordered four Ounces more to be taken in three or four Hours afterwards : The Pulfe rofe ftill more, and he ordered a Dofe of Sena and Rhubarb to be taken next Day, and the Patient recovered. And he adds, that all thofe who were treated in this manner got well. *Prax. Med. Lib.* XVII. *fect.* iii. *cap.* 1.

(*s*) Ibid.

(*t*) *Pringle's Obfervations on the Difeafes of the Army*, Part III. chap. vii

In

In *February* 1761, three Patients in the Decline of this Fever had Buboes formed in the
Groin, which proved critical. At firſt, on ob-
ſerving them, I ſuſpected them to be venereal;
but on examining the Patients, they obſtinately
denied their having any Reaſon to ſuſpect any
ſuch Cauſe; and the favourable Manner in
which they healed without the Appearance of
any other venereal Symptom, made me believe
what they aſſerted to be true ; eſpecially as ſuch
People are not ſhy in owning Complaints of
that Kind. The firſt Patient I ſaw who had a
Bubo in the Decline of one of theſe Malignant
Fevers, was a Woman, Wife to a Soldier of
the thirty-ſeventh Regiment of Foot; ſhe had
a Child at her Breaſt, and her Huſband was
living with her at the Time ſhe was taken ill
of the Fever, and neither of them had the leaſt
venereal Complaint. In a few Days afterwards,
two Soldiers in other Hoſpitals, towards the
Decline of very bad Petechial Fevers, had likewiſe Buboes formed in the Groin, without any
Suſpicion of a venereal Taint. Except in theſe
three, I did not ſee any critical Buboes appear
in this Fever while I was with the Troops in

Ger-

Germany; tho' Mr.*Lovet*, who ferved as a Mate
to the Hofpitals, and who was at *Hoxter*, where
we had another Hofpital eftablifh:d, while I
was at *Paderborn*, told me, that, in the Beginning of the Year 1761, they had feveral Men
in the Hofpital ill of this Fever, who had critical Buboes formed in the Groins and Arm-
pits (*u*).

About the fame Time that thefe Buboes appeared, feverals towards the Decline of this
Fever complained of a Pain all along the Sper-
matic Chord; and foon after a Swelling of the
Tefticle appeared (*x*). However, this Complaint was not peculiar to thofe who had the

(*u*) This Symptom of Buboes is taken Notice of by Authors, but does not feem to be fo frequent as many of them
would make us believe. Neither Dr. *Huxham* nor Dr. *Pringle*
mention their having feen fuch Buboes; and Dr. *Lind* fays,
that he never faw them till the Beginning of the Year 1763.

(*x*) *Hippocrates* takes Notice of Swellings of the Tefticles in
Fevers. He tells us, that a Man from Alcibiades had his left
Tefticle fwell before the Crifis of a Fever. *See his Second Book
on Epidemics*, fect. ii.   And he mentions this Symptom as a
Crifis in the ardent Fever. *See his Book on Crifes*, fect. xi. ——
And Dr. *Antonio Lizzari*, in a Treatife which he publifhed on
the *Acute Difeafes which were frequent at Venice, and all over
Italy, in the Years* 1761, 62, tells us, that Abfceffes of the
Scrotum and Tefticles frequently followed the Meafles.

Fever;

Fever; for others recovering from Fluxes, and other Diforders, were likewife affected with fuch Swellings. I did not obferve any Symptom of this Kind in Fevers while I was with the Troops in *Germany*, except in *January*, *February, March*, and *April* 1761. By Bleeding, and applying emollient Fomentations and Cataplafms, and bathing the Parts with *fpiritus mindereri* on the firft Attack of the Pain, the Swelling of the Tefticle was prevented; but where no Mention was made of this Pain till the Swelling had already begun, it commonly ended in a Suppuration of the Scrotum or Tefticle, which healed very kindly. We had no Reafon to fufpect any venereal Taint in any of them.

Many, while recovering from this Fever, were feized with an Ophthalmia, or Inflammation of the Eye; for the moft part of one Eye only, fometimes of both. When the Patients were ftrong, they were blooded, and had Blifters applied behind the Ears; and fometimes, where the Pain was great, had Poultices of Bread and Milk applied to the inflamed Eye; which, with the Affiftance of fome cooling Phyfic,

fick, commonly removed this Complaint; tho'
in fome obftinate Cafes we were obliged to repeat the Evacuations, to apply Leeches to the
Temples; and after the acute State of the Diforder was paffed, to order the Eye to be wafhed
frequently with the Collyrium vitriolicum, or
Collyrium Saturninum, before we got the better of this Complaint. However, it ought to
be obferved, that if thefe aftringent Collyria
were ufed too foon, they did hurt. When
thefe Ophthalmias were neglected in the Beginning, the Inflammation frequently rofe to a
great Height, and left an Obfcurity or Philm
over the Cornea, which remained an Impediment to the Sight not to be removed.

Towards the Decline of thefe Fevers, and very
often during the Courfe of them, many complained of Pains in their Feet and Toes, which
fometimes ended in Mortifications, efpecially
where the Patients lay in very cold Wards.
For the moft Part, the Mortification extended
no further than the Ends of the Toes, tho' in
fome it fpread over the Feet, and in two or
three advanced up the Leg. Several loft one

or

or more Toes ; and in *February* 1761, one
Man loft Half of each Foot ; another loft both
Feet, and Part of each Leg. Both got the better of the Fever, tho' the Man who loft both
Feet languifhed a long time afterwards. Thefe
Pains of the Feet and Toes, and the Mortifications which followed, were for the moft part
owing to the Patients being expofed to too
much Cold while they were very weak, the
Circulation languid, and the Juices vitiated by a
putrid Diftemper ; by which means the Veffels
were rendered incapable of carrying on the
Circulation in their extreme Branches (*y*).

As foon as the Sick began to complain of
thefe Pains of the Toes and Feet, I found the
beft Remedy to be, the Bathing of the Feet in

(*y*) Thefe Pains and Mortifications of the Feet and Toes
were not confined to thofe who were brought low by malignant
Fevers ; for, during the very hard Froft in the Beginning of
the Year 1763, many of the Patients who lay in very large
open Wards in the Hofpital at *Ofnabruck*, were affected in the
fame Way. One Man had both Feet, and Part of each Leg,
compleatly mortified, and died in about nine Days after the
firft Appearance of the Mortification. One loft half of one Foot,
and fome Toes of the other ; and the third loft the firft Joint of
fome of his Toes, and the Ends of others.

warm

warm Water, or in warm aromatic Fomentations; and, after keeping the Feet for some time
in these warm Liquors, to dry them well, and then
rub them with the *linimentum saponaceum*, or *linimentum volatile*, and wrap them up in Flannel.
And if ever any Lividness or Redness appeared
on the Parts, we gave plentifully of the Cortex
and Cordials, if not contra-indicated by the o-
ther Symptoms. When Vesicles arose on the
Part, and a Gangrene formed, we directed the
Parts to be scarified, and proper Dressings to be
applied, while warm aromatic Fomentations
and Cataplasms were used.

In *January* 1762, one Patient, ill of the
Petechial Fever at *Bremen*, had a Lividness and
Blackness, threatning a Mortification, which appeared at the End of his Nose. I expected for
some Days, that, if he recovered, he would lose
Part of his Nose; but, by giving him large and
repeated Doses of the *cortex* and *confectio cardiaca*, in a Mindereri Mixture, and allowing
him the free Use of Wine, its further Progress
was prevented; and as the Patient got clear of
the Fever, the Nose recovered its natural Colour,

lour, and only the fcarf Skin peeled off from the End of it.

When the Fever continued long, and reduced the Patients low, it was very common for the Back, and Parts on which the Weight of the Body refted, to mortify. As foon as any thing of this Kind was obferved, we ordered fuch Parts to be covered with proper Dreffings, and gave the Bark and Cordials freely; and took care to make the Patient change his Pofture; and by Pillows prevented as much as poffible the Weight of the Body from refting on that Part. By this Treatment, many recovered, where the Fever was on the Decline, and the Strength not too much exhaufted; even tho' a very large Surface of the Skin had mortified; but where the Patients were very low, and the Fever ftill continued, or where it was complicated with a Flux, which kept them perpetually nafty, and exhaufted the Strength, it generally proved fatal.

Patients, who were reduced very low by this Fever, or by repeated Relapfes, were fubject to oedematous Swellings; efpecially of the Feet,

E　　　　　　towards

towards the Evening, after fitting up all the Day.
Thefe Swellings generally went away as the
Sick recovered their Strength; but in fome
Cafes they continued obftinate, and afcended to-
wards the Thighs; and in fome fpread all over the
Body, and terminated in an univerfal Anafarca.

When thefe Swellings were recent, and confined to the Feet and Legs, commonly the
Bark joined to the lixivial Salts, or the Oxymel
of Squills, or other Diuretics, and a Purgative
once or twice a Week, removed them. In
fome, an Infufion of Horfe-radifh had a good
Effect; in others, Sweats brought out by
means of *Dover's* Powder, or of the *guttæ an-
timoniales anodynæ*.

 Sometimes thefe Swellings were very obftinate,
and refifted the Force of all internal Remedies.
In fuch Cafes, Punctures made in the Feet, or
lower Part of the Legs, which furnifhed a
Drain for the Water, had a good Effect. Blifters applied to the Legs were of Service to
fome. When the Punctures were made, or
the Blifters applied, before the Patient's
Strength was exhaufted, provided that he laboured

boured under no other Diforder but thefe oedematous Swellings, which proceeded from
Weaknefs, I never obferved any bad Effects
from them ; tho' I ufed them both repeatedly
in a Variety of Cafes. But if the Patient was
very weak ; or had a Hectic Fever or Purging;
or other Diforders, and the oedematous Swellings large ; then oftentimes the great Difcharge
exhaufted his Strength, and a Gangrene and
Death were the Confequence.

One of the moft remarkable Inftances of the
good Effects of Blifters ufed in this Way, was
in the Cafe of a Soldier at *Paderborn* ; *Thomas
Hope*, of the Second Regiment of Foot Guards,
after a Fever of this Kind, was fwelled all
over, efpecially about the Face and Neck,
and had a Difficulty of Breathing : after having tried Variety of Medicines for this Complaint, without any Effect, he had a large Blifter applied to his Back, and took the Cortex
in a Mixture, with the Oxymel of Squills.
As foon as the Blifter began to difcharge, the
Swellings decreafed; and were afterwards entirely removed by the Help of one or two Dofes

of

of Phyfic, and the continued Ufe of the Medicines before prefcribed. Three other Men in
the Hofpital at *Ofnabruck*, in *May* 1761, having oedematous Swellings of the Feet and Legs,
which yielded to no internal Remedies, had
Blifters applied to their Legs, ufed the Cortex,
with the lixivial Salts, two or three Times a
Day, and a Purge every fourth Day; which removed the Swellings in a fhort Time.

Some of the Soldiers, who had repeated
Hofpital Fevers, had their Blood fo much broke
down, as to be fubject to profufe Hæmor-
rhages from the Nofe; and fome of them paffed Blood likewife by Stool; which reduced
them to a very low State, fometimes attended
with imminent Danger. In fuch Cafes we
found nothing to anfwer fo well as to give
freely of the Bark; to acidulate their Drinks
with the *fpiritus vitrioli*; to allow them as
much Red Wine as the Strength and prefent
Circumftances could bear; and at the fame
Time to fupport the Patient's Strength by
a mild Diet, of light Digeftion; as Water or
Rice Gruel, Panado, weak Broth, and the
like.

like. When there was a Tendency to a Diarrhœa, we were obliged to add fome of the *electuarium diafcordii* to the Cortex, and frequently to give an Opiate in the Eveuing. One
Cafe, where this Method of Cure had a very
remarkable good Effect, l had under my Care
at *Paderborn*. A Soldier who lay in one of
the lower Wards of the Jefuits Hofpital, after
a Malignant Fever, attended with a Flux, ufed
to bleed at the Nofe, to four, five, or fix Ounces at a Time; and once or twice loft near a
Pint of Blood, of a dark Colour, very thin
and watery, and of fo loofe a Texture, that
the grumous Part fcarcely coagulated. This
Evacuation brought him fo low, that he could
fcarce turn himfelf in Bed; and his Pulfe
might be faid rather to flutter than beat:
By the continued Ufe of the Bark, and
of Cordials, and Drinks acidulated with *fpiritus vitrioli*, and fome Spoonfulls of mulled Red Wine every two or three Hours,
he was reftored to Health and Strength. The
only Accident which happened during the
Cure, was a Threatening of a Loofenefs, and the
Return of his Flux; which however was ftopt

E 3   by

by a Dofe of the *tinctura rhei*; by joining fome of the *electuarium diafcordii* with the Bark, and giving an Opiate in the Evening.

Putrid Malignant Fevers, attended with Eruptions, are taken Notice of by *Hippocrates* (*z*), and other antient Authors (*a*); but whether they meant that particular Sort of Eruption which we now call Petechiæ, is uncertain; as their Defcriptions are not clear enough to diftinguifh it from the Miliary and other Kinds. But fince the Year 1500, we have had many accurate Accounts of Fevers of this Kind, which have appeared in different Parts of the World: from all which 'it appears that fuch Fevers generally take their Rife either from fome antecedent Acrimony of the Blood; or, what is more frequent, from fome Source of Corruption or Contagion; from the Ufe of putrefcent animal Food, and a Want of frefh Vegetables and acefcent Liquors; from

(*z*) *Hippocrat.* lib. ii. popul. fect. iii. text. 2.

(*a*) *Aetius Tetrab.* ii. fect. i. cap. 129.   *Actuar.* lib. i. cap. 23.

the

the putrid Steams of corrupted animal Subftances ; from the moift putrid Vapour of low
marfhy Places in Summer, where there is ftagnating Water, which corrupts by the Heat;
from the foul Air of crowded Hofpitals, Jails,
and Ships ; and from fuch like Caufes (*b*).

When once this Fever begins, it is obferved
to be of a contagious Nature, and (if proper
Care is not taken) to affect thofe who attend
the Sick, or who live in the fame Room, and
breathe the fame Air with them.

Many Authors have reckoned the Malignant, Petechial, and Peftilential, to be diftinct
Species of Fevers; and have treated each of
them under a particular Head. But *Riverius* (*c*) has very juftly obferved, that they all
belong to the fame peftilential Tribe, and only
differ from one another in the Degree of In-

(*b*) See thefe Caufes mentioned by *Riverius*, and fince more
fuily explained by Dr. *Pringle*, *Obfervations on the Difeafes of
the Army*, part iii. chap. vii.

(*c*) *River. Prax. Med.* lib. xvi. fect. iii. Præfat.

E 4   fection,

fection, and the Violence of the Symptoms (*d*);
and that they are to be cured by the fame general Treatment, and the fame Medicines.

(*d*) The Malignant or Hofpital Fever, and Petechial, feemed
to me to be entirely the fame Diforder, and the Petechial Spots
to be only a Symptom which appeared fometimes, but not always. And *Riverius* fays, the Petechiæ do not always appear;
but when they do, it is a moft certain Sign of a Peftilential Fever. See his *Prax. Med.* cap. xvi. feft. iii.

O F

OF THE

DYSENTERY.

THE Dyfentery generally began to appear foon after the Army took the Field; and became frequent about the End of *July*, and continued fo till the Army went into Winter-Quarters; and through the Winter, many of thofe, who had this Diforder in Autumn, relapfed, upon returning to their Duty; or by drinking too freely of fpirituous Liquors, and being irregular in their Living.

It is now generally agreed upon, that this Diforder is entirely produced by fuch Caufes as make the Juices become too putrefcent, and turn the Flow of Humours to the Bowels; and in the Camp it feemed to arife principally from an obftruded Perfpiration caufed by the Men's lying

lying in the Field, and doing the neceffary Military Duties in all Sorts of Weather ; at the fame Time being often expofed to the putrid Steams of dead Horfes, of the Privies, and of other corrupted Animal or Vegetable Subftances (*a*), after their Juices had been highly exalted by the Heat of Summer.

At

(*a*) The Dyfentery has been long alledged to arife from a putrefcent Caufe in Camps ; from the Smell of corrupted dead Animals, and of Excrements, during the Heat of Summer. *Ramazzini*, in his Chapter on Camp-Difeafes, informs us, that Dr. G. *Erric Barnftorff*, Phyfician to the Duke of *Brunfwick*, who ferved five Campaigns with the *Brunfwick* and *Lunenburg* Troops in *Hungary*, told him, that the Camp-Difcafes, particularly the Malignant Fever and Dyfentery, took their Rife from the Troops remaining long encamped on the fame Ground, and being expofed to the corrupted Steams of the Bodies of dead Men, Horfes, and other Animals, which lay unburied ; and of Excrements, which were not covered with Earth. And thefe Caufes have fince been particularly taken notice of by Dr. *Pringle*, in his *Obfervations on the Difeafes of the Army.*

Many have imputed the Caufe of this Diforder to the eating of Fruit in excefs, becaufe it geneially appears about the Middle of Summer, the Time the Fruit begins to be in Seafon, and continues through the Autumn. But from later Obfervations this fhould feem to be a vulgar Error. Dr. *Pringle*

(part

At the Time the Petechial Fever was frequent at *Paderborn* in *January*, *February*, and
March 1761, the Flux frequently accompanied
it;

(part i. ch. iii. p. 20.) tells us, that, in the Year 1743, this
Sickness began and raged before any Fruit was in Season, except Strawberries, (which from their high Price the Men never
tasted) and ended about the Time the Grapes were ripe; which
growing in open Vineyards were freely eat by every body.
And Dr. *Tissot*, in a Treatise which he published, called *Avis
au Peuple sur la Santé*, in his Chapter on the *Dysentery*, § 320,
says, that ripe Fruit, especially the Summer-Fruits, are so far
from being the Cause of the Disorder, that they are the great
Preservatives against it: he says, that, in the Years which the
Fruit is most plentiful, the Dysentery is least frequent; and
he relates several Instances where the Use of ripe Grapes proved a Cure for the Disorder. Eleven People were attacked by
the Dysentery, nine eat Fruit, and all recovered; the other
two, a Grandmother and Child, from Prejudice, eat none,
and both died. A Regiment of *Swiss* Soldiers, in Garrison in
the South of *France*, had the Dysentery very frequent among
them. The Captains purchased some Acres of a Vineyard, and
carried the sick Soldiers to the Field, and gave them the
Grapes to eat; and ordered the Men in Health to live upon
them chiefly. After this not one Person died, nor was any
one seized with the Distemper. — In an Account of a Treatise
on the Dysentery, published at *Hamburg* in 1753, which was
epidemical the Year before, in *August* and *September*, we are
told, that it did not proceed, as is commonly believed, from
the eating of Fruit; for it was observed, that those who eat

it; and we had in the Hofpitals likewife a Number of old Cafes of this Kind, the Remains of the preceding Campaign about *Warbourg*; befides fome Men who had relapfed during the Winter, and were fent to us when the Troops marched, upon the Winter-Expedition, into the Country of *Heſſe*. In *May* and *June*, what Fluxes we had at *Ofnabruck*, were the remaining old Cafes of the Hofpitals of *Munſter*, *Paderborn*, *Hoxter*, and *Niehms*. Some few recent ones were fent to *Bilifield* about the End of *June*, and above 300 to *Munſter*, in *July* and *Auguſt*. Thofe fent to *Bremen*, in *November* and *December*, had continued for fome time before they reached us; but a good many of the Soldiers in the Garrifon were taken ill of this Diforder, and fent immediately to the Hofpital. In the

Fruit freely efcaped better than thofe who abſtained from it altogether. *Vide Comment. de Rebus in Hiſt. Nat. & Medecin. Geſtis,* vol. II. par. iv. feʤ. v.

Generally in *Auguſt* and *September* we have People admitted into *St. George*'s Hofpital for the Dyfentery; who have certainly not catched the Diforder from eating of Fruit, but from working in the Fields, and being expofed to Caufes fimilar to thofe which produce the Dyfentery in Camps.

Beginning

Beginning of *May* we had but four ill of this Complaint in the Hofpital I attended; and there were not above fix or feven, among the Sick fent down from the Army, in the Middle of this Month. In *June* there were but two fent to the Hofpital at *Minden*; and not above ten among the Sick fent to *Natzungen* in the Beginning of *July*; tho' towards the Middle of this Month they began to be more frequent; and continued to be more fo in *Auguft* and *September*; and in the Hofpital at *Ofnabruck* we had not above five or fix ill of this Diforder, in *December* 1762, and in *January*, *February* and *March* 1763.

The Dyfentery commonly begun with Sicknefs and Gripes, fucceeded by a Purging, and attended with more or lefs Fever. Very foon the Gripes became more fevere, attended with a Flatulency in the Bowels, and often with a Tenefmus. The Stools were chiefly compofed of Mucus, mixed with Bile, and more or lefs Blood : tho' fometimes no Blood could be obferved in them ; and then the Soldiers ufed to fay they had the White Flux.

After

After eight, ten, or twelve, Days, if the Diſorder was not complicated with any other, there remained little or no Fever, unleſs where ſome Accident ſupervened ; tho' in Caſes which terminated fatally, towards the latter End came on a Fever of a low malignant Kind, attended with black fetid Stools, Lientery, Hiccup, Stupor, and other bad Symptoms.

It often happened, that, after the Dyſentery had continued for ſome Time, the Sick complained for a Day or two of ſevere Gripes ; and then diſcharged along with the Stools little Pieces of hardened Excrements ; at other Times, tho' more rarely, little Pieces of white Stuff like Tallow or Suet : Frequently ſmall Filaments, and little Pieces of Membranes, were found floating in the Stools; and it was very common for the Sick to vomit up Worms of the round Kind, or diſcharge them by Stool *(b)*.

In the Courſe of the Diſorder, the Men often complained of a violent Pain of the Rectum,

(*b*) Moſt Authors, who treat of the Dyſentery, mention this Symptom of Worms ; and Dr. *Huxham* tells us, that, in ſome Seaſons, he has ſeen round Worms in the Stools of moſt of the Dyſenteric Patients. *De Aëre,* vol. II. p. 98.

near

near the Fundament, which was moſt excrucia-
ting when they went to Stool; it continued for
ſome Days, ſometimes for a Week or more; and
then they paſſed more or leſs of a Yellow Pus
with their Excrements, and the violent Pain
ceaſed. Mr. *A. Tough*, one of the Apothecaries to
the Military Hoſpital in *Germany*, was the firſt
who told me that I ſhould find Pus mixed with
the Stools: on my mentioning a Caſe of this
Kind, which had been relieved by Bleeding,
and Clyſters often repeated ; he told me he had
obſerved it frequently at *Gibraltar* ; and was at
a Loſs to underſtand the Nature of the Symptom, till he obſerved the Matter in the Stools;
which at once ſhewed him that it had been originally an acute Inflammation of the Part, and
pointed out to him the proper Method of
Cure.

Oftentimes the Bilious and Malignant Fevers
terminated in the Dyſentery; or were accompanied with it, when it might be looked upon as a
Symptom of theſe Fevers.

The Appearances we found after Death in the
Bodies of ſome Patients, who died of old Fluxes

at

at *Bremen*, were : In all of them the Rectum was inflamed, and partly gangrened, efpecially the internal Coat. In two the lower Part of the Colon was inflamed, and there were feveral livid Spots on its great Arcade. In one whofe Body was much emaciated, and who had been feized with a violent Pain of the Bowels two Days before his Death, all the fmall Guts were red and inflamed ; and in another there were livid gangrened Spots on the Stomach(*c*).

There was no Diforder we were more fuccefsful in the Cure of,. than recent Fluxes ; but after they had continued for Weeks, and were become in a manner chronic, they often foiled all

our

(*c*) From the Accounts we have in Authors, of the Diffection of the Bodies of Perfons who died of the Dyfentery, it would appear ; that there is no Part of the alimentary Canal which has not fome time or other been found inflamed, or in a ftate of Suppuration or Gangrene ; and the Liver, Spleen, and other Vifcera, have likewife been found difeafed, but the Rectum and Colon have almoft in all been more or lefs affected. The following Account I had, in the Year 1748, from the late Dr. *L. Frafer*, who afterwards practifed in the Ifland of *Nevis*, two Days after the Patient died. *Mary Reid*, a Woman thirty Years of Age, was taken ill of a Dyfentery, which in Three

Weeks

our Endeavours, and a great Number died (*d*).

Weeks Time killed her. In her Life-time she complained, more than ordinary, of Gripes in her Belly, especially in her Left Side. Her Body was opened in Presence of Dr. *Dundas*, who had attended her, during her Illness. All the Intestines and Mesentery were inflamed, especially the Colon and Rectum ; the internal Side of which was quite in a mortified State, and contained little Vesicles full of a putrid fetid Liquor, Numbers of which she had evacuated by Stool some Days before her Death.

While this Sheet was in the Press, I received Dr. *Pringle*'s 4th Edition of his *Observations on the Diseases of the Army*, and Dr. *Baker*'s Treatise on the *Dysentery which was epidemic in London in the Year* 1762. Both these Gentlemen give an Account of the Dissection of the Bodies of some People who died of the Dysentery ; where, besides the common Appearances of the inner Surface of the Rectum and Colon being covered with a bloody Slime, and their internal Coats being inflamed, gangrened, or in a putrid State, there were observed on the Inside of the lower Part of the Colon, and upper Part of the Rectum, a Number of little Tubercles, or Excrescences, which resembled the Small Pox, of a flat Sort at the Height of the Disorder ; but differed from them in this, that they were of a firm Consistence, without any Cavity : they were believed to take their Rise from the cellular Membrane, which lies immediately above the villous Coat. Perhaps such Tubercles might have been found in the Colon and Rectum of those Bodies we opened ; but not looking for them, they may have passed unobserved. '

Morgagni, in his Book lately published, *de Sede & Causis Morborum*, epist. xxxi. is of Opinion, that the Filaments, and Pieces of Membranes, which are frequently observed in the Stools, are often formed of inspissated Mucus and Lymph, and other Liquors; and not the Fibres, or Pieces of the villous Coat of the Intestines, as alledged by many Authors.

F   Upon

Upon my firſt being employed in the Military
Hoſpitals in *Germany*, I was ſurpriſed to ſee ſo
many of the old Dyſenteric Caſes end fatally;
and imagined I had not fallen upon the Right
Method of treating them : but upon conſulting
the other Phyſical People employed in the ſame
Service, I found them as unſucceſsful, as myſelf,
after having tried a Variety of Remedies : And
at laſt, I was convinced, that when once the Flux
had continued long, and injured the Structure of
the Inteſtines to a certain Length, a Gangrene

(*d*) Mr. *Cleghorn*, in his *Account of the Diſeaſes of the Iſland of
Minorca*, ſays, " That almoſt all the Dyſenteries which fell un-
" der my Obſervation, unleſs they were ſpeedily cured in the
" Beginning, at beſt proved obſtinate, and too frequently fatal,
" in ſpite of the many boaſted Specificks for this Diſtemper."
chap. v. p. 228. — The phyſical Gentlemen employed on the
American Service have told me, that the old Flux Caſes were
as fatal in *America,* as we found them in *Germany.* I would not
from thence have it believed, that every old Flux was to be
looked on as a loſt Caſe ; and for that Reaſon given up, and no
Attempts be made to cure it; for many, by great Care, and
Strength of Conſtitution, have gradually ſurmounted the Diſorder, and recovered their Health ; eſpecially when they got over
the Winter, and lived till the warm Weather began.

will

will often form by flow Degrees; and the Diforder end fatally, notwithftanding the Ufe of what
are efteemed the moft efficacious Remedies; and
that, when this Diforder is violent, the Cure
principally depends upon an early and fpeedy
Application of proper Remedies, before the
Strength be exhaufted, or the Structure of the
Bowels too much hurt. The bad Succefs we
had in treating thefe old Cafes, may perhaps
furprife thofe who have never practifed except
in healthful Cities, where the Difeafe is commonly mild, and People apply foon for Advice. But all thofe Gentlemen who have had
the Care of Military Hofpitals, where the Dyfentery has been frequent, and where the Sick
have been often fent a great Way, before they
reached the Hofpitals, muft be convinced of the
Truth of what is here afferted.

In the Treatment of this Diforder, as well as
of the Malignant Fever, nothing contributed
more to the Cure, than keeping the Sick as
clean as poffible, and in large airy Wards.

F 2 Moft

Moſt of the recent Fluxes, which I ſaw, were at firſt attended with a good deal of Fever, and Pain in the Bowels; and required more or leſs Blood to be taken away, according to the Strength of the Patient, and the Violence of the Symptoms.

When the Patients were ſtrong, and com-plained of ſharp Pain of the Bowels, attended with a Fever, we uſed the Lancet freely; nor were we diſcouraged from bleeding in the Beginning by the low quick Pulſe which ofteñ attended the Diſorder; and we frequently found the Pulſe riſe as the Blood flowed from the Vein. But when the Sick were low and weak, without much Pain or Fever, and the Pulſe was ſoft, we were more ſparing of the vital Fluid (*e*).

As

(*e*) Although Bleeding, in the Beginning, has been recom-mended by *Sydenham*, *Huxham*, *Pringle*, and other Practitioners; yet it has been reckoned unneceſſary in this Diſorder by ſome late Authors. But in moſt of the recent Caſes I ſaw, it was ex-tremeſy neceſſary, and contributed greatly to the Relief as

well

As the Diforder was for the moft part attended with Sicknefs in the Beginning, we gave a Vomit after bleeding; which not only difcharged the Contents .of the Stomach, and a Quantity of Bile, but relieved the Sicknefs, and frequently threw the Patient into a breathing Sweat; and made the Purgatives which were given next Day operate more freely, and with more evident good Effects than where no Vomit had been adminiftered.—If in the Courfe of the Difeafe the Sicknefs returned, the Emetic was repeated; and we often obferved, when the Flux was obftinate, that well-timed Vomits

well as the Cure of the Patient; indeed where the Diforder had already continued fome time, and the Fever was gone off before the Patient was fent to us; and the Diforder had become in a manner chronic, and the Patient low, then bleeding was unneceffary, and would have probably done Hurt. Mr. *Francis Ruffel* told me, that when the Dyfentery was epidemical at *Gibraltar*, in Summer 1756, he found that by bleeding fuch Patients as he met with at the firft coming on of the Symptoms, and by giving them immediately a Vomit, and afterwards a fudorific Draught, the Diforder was rendered mild, and few of thofe died.

greatly

greatly promoted the Cure.—The Vomit we commonly employed was the Powder of Ipecacuana, which we gave from ten to twenty Grains; and where the Patient was ftrong, and we wanted to make a free Evacuation, we added one, two, or three Grains of the Tartar Emetic; which encreafed the Strength of the Vomit, and commonly operated likewife by Stool (*f*), as Dr. *Pringle* has obferved.

Next Day we ordered a Purge to empty the other Parts of the alimentary Canal. The Purgative, that at firft was moft employed for this Purpofe, was Rhubarb; but upon repeated Trials we did not find, that, in general, it anfwered fo well, in this firft Stage of the Diforder, as the *fal catharticum amarum,* with Manna

(*f*) Mr. *W. Ruffel,* who was with the Hofpital at *Martinico,* told me, that, when he was there, he found the Vomit with the Tartar Emetic to be far preferable to any other, in all Cafes where there was much putrid Bile lodged in the alimentary Canal; as it fpeedily carried off thofe corrupt Humours, which were often productive of the greateft Mifchiefs, if they remained, but for a fhort Time, pent up within the Bowels.

and

and Oil; which operated without griping or disturbing the Patient, procured a freer Evacuation, and gave greater Relief than any other purgative Medicine we tried. Mr. *Francis Ruffel*, Surgeon to the *British* Military Hospital in *America*, who was formerly Surgeon to the Island of *Minorca*, was the first Person who informed me (in the Year 1757) of the Use of the *fal cathar-ticum amarum* in the Dysentery; he told me, that the Year before (1756) the Dysentery had been very frequent and very fatal at *Gibraltar*; and, after trying Variety of Medicines, he had found nothing give more Relief, or contribute more to the Cure, than repeated Doses of these Salts.

As a great Part of the Cure depended on the frequent Use of gentle Purges (*g*) in the Beginning

(*g*) Variety of Medicines have been recommended to answer this Purpose.

The *vitrum ceratum antimonii* proved often too rough a Medicine, and therefore we laid it almost entirely aside.

Repeated small Doses of the Ipecacuana, from four to six

ning, to carry off the corrupted Humours; the
Purgative was repeated every fecond, third, or
fourth Day, as the Cafe required; the Operation

Grains, operated both as an Emetic, and kept up a Purging;
but they made the Men fo fick, that we could not prevail upon
them to continue their Ufe. Mr. *Francis Ruffel* told me, that,
in the Year 1756, he found a few Grains of Rhubarb added
to each Dofe, made it operate more as a Purgative, and did
not make the Men fo fick.——Dr. *Akenfide* propofes giving the
Ipecacuana in fo fmall Dofes as one or two Grains every fix
Hours, in a Draught made of Mint-water, and Half a Drachm
of *confectio cardiaca*; and, after bleeding and vomiting once,
feems to depend almoft entirely on the Ufe of this Medicine for
the Cure of the Dyfentery. See his *Comment. de Dyfenteria,*
cap. 2.

The watery Tincture of Rhubarb, recommended by *Degnerus*, we tried in fome Cafes at Bremen; and found it to be a
good mild Purge, but not to anfwer fo well as the Salts and
Manna in recent Cafes. Mr. *William Ruffel* told me that they
found this watery Tincture of Rhubarb to anfwer better in
America than any other of the Preparations of Rhubarb.

Calomel has been recommended by many as a Purge in Dyfenteries; and Dr. *Huxham* (*de Aere*, Vol. II. P. 100) affures
us, that he has often experienced the good Effects of it, efpecially when the Patient at the fame time had Worms; in fuch
Cafes we joined it to Rhubarb as mentioned in the Text, or
gave a Calomel Bolus over Night, and a Purge next Morning.

Dr. -

tion of the former Purge, and the Symptoms, determining the Frequency of the Repetition. It

Dr. *Duncan*, Phyfician to his Majefty, told me, that he found the following Method of Cure always fuccefsful in the Dyfentery, which was epidemic in *London* in the Year 1762.

If the Patient was Plethoric, or had much Fever, he ordered more or lefs Blood to be taken away; and then gave four Ounces of the following Julep, every Half Hour, till it both vomited and purged. R *Tartar. emetic. gr.* iij *Mannæ elect. Unc.* ij *folve in Aq. hordeat. Lib.* 1.——The next Day, and for five or fix Days more, the Patient took fo much of a Decoction, of Manna, Tamarinds, and foluble Tartar, as kept up a free Difcharge by Stool.—If the Irritation and Griping were fevere, he found that a Solution of Manna, in the common Almond Emulfion, was fufficient.

When the Pain, or Tenefmus, was violent, a Clyfter, of Chicken Broth, or of an Infufion of Linfeed, with an Ounce or two of Oil of fweet Almonds diffolved in the Yolk of an Egg, injected once or twice a Day, was of great Ufe.

Upon the whole, he was always pleafed when he faw large excrementitious Stools come away; and when that could be procured by a gentle Method, he was the more pleafed.

This Diforder was very often cured in a few Days, and in that Cafe he dropt the further Ufe of Medicines; but when it exceeded the Period of fix or feven Days, he then added thirty or forty Drops of the *tinctura thebaica* to the Clyfters; and ordered a Scruple of the Extract of the Logwood to be taken thrice a Day in fome proper Vehicle.

The Patient's Diet was Rice-Gruel, Sago, Panado, and fuch like; no Animal Food, not fo much as Chicken-Broth, was

allowed

It was furprifing with how little Lofs of Strength
the Sick bore the Operation of thefe Purges; I
have fometimes given them to ftrong People

allowed in the Beginning of the Diftemper, nor even Oil, Butter, or Fat of any Kind. The common Drink was Almond
Emulfion, Rice-Water, or Barley-Water with Gum Arabic.

Dr. *Duncan* loft but one Patient out of Eighty, whom he had
under his Care that Seafon ; and he was delirious, had a high
Fever, and a *fubfultus tendinum* before the Doctor was called
to him, and he died the next Day.

The late Dr. *Young*, of *Edinburgh*, feems to have had a very
juft Notion of this Diforder, and of the proper Method of
treating it ; for, in his Treatife on Opium, fect. vii. he fays,
" I am convinced from Experience, that moft of the Dyfente-
" ries I have hitherto met with, might have been cured by
" purging mildly, but conftantly ; and at the fame time abating
" the Acrimony in the great Guts by emollient Clyfters, and
" in the fmall ones by Plenty of Abforbents, and a Diet of
" Chicken Broth : But it muft be obferved with regard to Pur-
" gatives, that Manna agrees beft with fome, Rhubarb with
" others, Jalap, Mercury, and toafted Rhubarb with others ;
" while others are fooner cured by emollient Clyfters. I ufe
" Opium only when the Difeafe is mild, or after its Violence is
" abated by Evacuants and Emollients."

Scammony, Aloes, and the other ftrong refinous and hydragogue
Purges, are hurtful, and occafion Pain. I always obferved, that
thofe Purges anfwered beft which made the freeft Evacuation,
and acted with the greateft Eafe to the Patient ; of which the
Salts and Manna anfwered beft of any I have hitherto ufed."

every

every Day, for two, three, or four Days fucceffively; and obferved that the Patient, inftead
of being weakened, feemed ftronger, and more
brifk and lively, after the Operation of each,
from the Relief it gave; by evacuating thofe
putrid, corrupted Humours, which kept him
perpetually fick and uneafy, while they remained within the Bowels.

Though Rhubarb did not anfwer fo well in
the Beginning as the faline Purges; yet afterwards in the Courfe of the Diftemper, when
the Patient did not complain much of Gripes,
half a Drachm of Rhubarb, either by itfelf or
in a faline Draught, proved a good gentle
Purge; and given with fix or feven Grains of
Calomel, was found to be a good Medicine,
when the Diforder was attended with Worms.

In the Evening, after the Operation of the
Purge, we gave an Opiate; and repeated it at
Nights, in the Intervals between the Purges;
but were obliged to be very fparing of the Dofe,
while the Diforder continued in its acute State;
the Opiate was only given in a Quantity fuffi-
çient to mitigate the Pain, and to procure Reft,
but

but never fo as to ftupify the Patient, or prevent a due Difcharge by Stool; though we were often obliged to encreafe the Dofe, as Ufe made it familiar to the Patient.

In the Intervals between the Purges, we gave in the Day, the Mindereri Draughts with the Mithridate; or the faline Draughts with the Addition of four Drops of the *tinctura the-baica*; or fome fuch mild diaphoretic, every four or fix Hours; which helped to keep up a free Perfpiration, without any Danger of ftopping the Purging; and for the moft part anfwered much better than the Diafcord, or Philonium, or other ftrong Aftringents and Opiates commonly prefcribed for this Purpofe; which were always liable to check the Purging too much, and bring on fevere Gripes attended with Heat and Fever (*h*); and therefore we feldom made Ufe of them in this firft Stage of the Diforder.

(*h*) *Sydenham, Huxham,* and all good Practitioners, have taken Notice of the bad Effects of the too free Ufe of Aftringents, and given Cautions againft it.

If

If the Patient was attacked with fevere Gripes (*i*), and a Tenefmus, which the Purgatives and gentle Opiates did not relieve, we ordered the Abdomen to be fomented with warm Stupes; and the Patient to drink freely of warm Barley or Rice-water, or of weak Broth (*k*), or an Infufion of Camomile Flowers, as recommended by Dr. *Pringle* ; and ordered firft Clyfters of large Quantities of the plain emollient Decoction to be given; and if the Gripes ftill

(*i*) If the Patient was fuddenly attacked with fharp Pain of the Bowels and Gripes, on a Day in which he had not Phyfic, a Dofe of the Salts and Manna was commonly given immediately, to empty thoroughly the firft Paffages.

(*k*) Mr. *W.Ruffel* told me, that he and Dr. *Huck* found the free Ufe of the following Emulfion, made of BeesWax, to be of great Ufe after Evacuations, where there was much Pain of the Bowels, in recent Cafes of Fluxes in the Hofpitals in *America*. R. Ceræ alb. vel flavæ drachmes tres. Sapon. alb. Hifpan. drachmam unam. Aquæ fontanæ, unciam unam, liquefiant fuper ignem in vafe ferreo, agitando fpatula, & dein infunde in mortarium marmoreum, & adde paulatim aq. fontanæ, libras duas fyrupi facchari. fpiritus vini gallici tenuis, vel aquæ alicujus fpirituofæ ana unciam unam, terendo optime ut fiat emulfio.

This Method of diffolving Bees Wax, in a Watery Liquor, is entirely new; for before this we knew of no Way of making it mifcible with Water.

conti-

continued, to be repeated in fmall Quantities, with the Addition of a Drachm or two of the *tinctura thebaica*; for we obferved that Opiate Clyfters often gave more Relief, than Anodynes adminiftered in any other Way; and fometimes, when a Tenefmus was very troublefome, the common oily Clyfter, with a little Diafcord, and *tinctura thebaica*, or the Starch Clyfter, gave more Eafe than any other.——In fome Cafes, where the Pain was fharp, attended with a Fever, we were obliged to take away more or lefs Blood; and fometimes alfo to apply a Blifter to that Part of the Abdomen where the Patient felt moft Pain.

During this Courfe, the Patients ufed the common low Diet of the Hofpital; when they loathed the Rice-Gruel, they had Panado with a little Red Wine and Sugar; or Water-gruel, when it could be got, in its Place.——Their common Drink was Barley or Rice-water; of which it was recommended to them to drink plentifully; as nothing contributed more to the Cure than the free Ufe of fuch Liquors, to dilute

and

and blunt the Acrimony of the Fluids (*l*). In some Cafes, when the Purging was violent, and not accompanied with the malignant Fever, the *decoctum album* was found to be a good Drink ; and we added occafionally a few Drops of the *tinctura thebaica*.

Such were the chief Remedies we ufed in the firft Stage of this Diforder; but after fome Weeks, when the Fever had abated, and free Evacuations had been made, and the Complaint become in a manner chronic, we were obliged to try other Methods ; and found that the beft Way of treating this Diforder, was, to endeavour to brace and reftore the Tone of the Inteftines, by means of the corroborating and gentle aftringent Medicines, mixed with Opiates;

(*l*) Dr. *Huxham* (*de Aere*, Vol. II. p. 107.) fays, there is no Diforder in which a diluting, fweetening Drink is more neceffary than in this; that he has done great Service among the Poor by luke-warm Water ; that, after emptying the Bowels thoroughly, he has fometimes cured this Diforder by the Ufe of pure Water, and a fmall Quantity of Opium. And *Baglivi* (*Prax. Med.* lib. i.) tells us, that the drinking of common Whey, and throwing up frequent Clyfters of it, had cured many, and that this was looked upon as a Specific, and kept a Secret by fome.

while

while mild Purgatives were given at proper Intervals.

The Patients were kept to the fame low Diet as before, with the Addition of a little Wine or Brandy. They were allowed from a Gill to a Pint of red Wine *per* Day, which was commonly mulled before it was given them ; when the Wine griped them, which it frequently did, they took in its Stead Half a Gill or a Gill of Brandy, mixed with a Pint or a Quart of Barley or Rice-water, or of the *decoctum album.*

In this Stage of the Diforder we found, that the fame Medicines would not anfwer with all, and therefore we were obliged to try Variety (*m*);

and

(*m*) Dr. *Pringle,* in the *fourth Edition of his Obfervations,* juft publifhed, in treating of the third or laft Stage of the Dyfentery, remarks, that this is the Time for Aftringents, which ought not to be given fooner, or at leaft very fparingly. And he tells us, that, in the former Editions of his Work, he mentioned thofe Compofitions which he had moft frequently ufed, but that he had now laid moft of them afide ; and at prefent trufts to Vomits, and to a Milk Diet, for the perfect Cure.

He fays, " Whenever therefore the Patient is in this State, " and efpecially when his Pulfe is quick, and he complains of " inward

and indeed, unlefs where the Violence of the
Diforder had abated by the Ufe of Evacuations,
the Event was always very doubtful; for when
the Complaint had continued long and become
chronic, and the Structure of the Inteftines
was much hurt, before the Sick were fent to us;
or when it continued obftinate, and yielded but
little to Evacuations, and the other Methods
ufed in the firft Stage, even Remedies efteemed

" inward Heat, I began with giving him a Scruple of Ipecacu-
" ana; and the next Day I put him upon the Milk-Diet; which
" I continue till all the hectic Symptoms are gone, and till the
" Bowels have recovered their Tone. During this Courfe I
" have feldom had Occafion for any other Medicine, excepting
" the Chalk Julep mentioned before, which I ufe for correcting
" that ftrong Acid fo incident to relaxed Stomachs. Some-
" times alfo I add an Opiate to procure Reft at Night; but after
" a few Days thefe are likewife laid afide. All that I require
" (which indeed is often hard to obtain) is a ftrict Perfeverance
" in the low Diet: and now and then a Repetition of the Vomit,
" upon any new Diforder of the Stomach, or great Laxity of
" the Bowels.

" Whilft the Patient continues in this Courfe, I forbid all a-
" nimal Food and fermented Liquors; and befides Milk, I al-
" low only the Preparations of Grain, Sago and Salop." See
Part iii. ch. vi. p. 289, 290.

G   the

the moſt efficacious oftentimes proved unſucceſsful, and at length the Patient died.

A Spoonful of the *mixtura fracaſtorii*, taken
after every looſe Stool; and an anodyne Draught
at Night, had a good Effect with ſome——Repeated Doſes of the *philonium Londinenſe* anſwered better with others, who were low, and
required a Remedy that was warm and cordial
——And others found more Benefit from the
Mindereri Draughts, with Mithridate, or the
confectio cardiaca, or theTheriac anodyne Boluſes.

The *mixtura Campechenſis*, both alone and
with *tinctura thebaica*, checked the Purging,
and gave Relief ſometimes; and the Addition
of ſome of the Extract of Bark and Tincture
of Cinnamon, ſeemed to encreaſe its Efficacy in
one or two old Caſes, at *Bremen*; but it afterwards occaſioned ſuch Sickneſs, that we did not
continue its Uſe.

In other inveterate Dyſenteries, where we
thought that a ſtrong Aſtringent was wanted,
we added a ſmall Proportion of Allum to the
Campechenſe Julep, which on firſt uſing ſeemed

to

to be ferviceable; but at other Times it occafioned a Tenefmus and Gripes; and therefore we were obliged to be very cautious how we ufed it.

Equal Parts of the *electuarium diafcordii* and *electuarium corticis,* taken in the Quantity of a Drachm twice or thrice a Day, was of Ufe in many old Fluxes (*n*), though it made other Patients fo fick, that they were obliged to lay it afide.

We tried likewife in this Stage of the Diforder, repeated fmall Dofes of the Ipecacuana; but it occafioned fuch Sicknefs, that we did not perfift in its Ufe.

(*n*) I had lately a very remarkable Inftance of the Effects of this Medicine, in the Cafe of one *Gilchrift,* a middle-aged Man; by Trade a Taylor; who was admitted into *St. George*'s Hofpital the 20th of *July,* 1763, for an old Flux, which had continued above fix Months, and reduced him very low: He had taken a great many Medicines without any Effect. After giving him a Vomit and two Dofes of Tincture of Rhubarb, I gave him four Grains of the Powder of Ipecacuana with Opium three Times a Day; but that having no Effect, after ufing it for above a Fortnight, I ordered him the Electuary of Diafcord and Cortex; from the Time he began to ufe this Medicine, he mended daily; and was difmiffed in good Health the 26th of *September.*

G 2   In

In other Cafes, we gave from two to five
Grains of the Ipecacuana, mixed with Opium,
in different Proportions (from three Grains to
ten of the Ipecacuana to one of the Opium),
every four or fix Hours; it gave fometimes a
little prefent Eafe, at other Times it occafioned
Sicknefs; we often continued its Ufe for ten,
twelve, or fourteen Days; but it feldom produced any remarkable Change for the better,
and we were obliged to have Recourfe to other
Remedies.   -

Dover's Powder was given in large Dofes,
from one Scruple to two; and proved a good
Sudorific and Anodyne in fome Cafes; though
in others it made the Patients fick, without
producing any good Effect.—It commonly anfwered better, when ufed occafionally as a Sudorific, than when conftantly continued.

During the Ufe of thefe Remedies, it was
neceffary to repeat the Purgatives from Time to
Time; or to mix them occafionally with the
other Medicines, in order to carry off any corrupted Humours, or Excrements that might
be lodged in the Cavity of the Inteftines; for
when

when this was neglected, the Patients were often 'feized with Sicknefs and Gripes, and a more violent Purging than before :—And if at any Time they complained of Gripes, and paffed little Pieces of hardened Excrements, it was moftly a certain Sign that a Purge was indicated ; and, on fuch Occafions, it generally gave Relief ; and when attended with Sicknefs, a Vomit was given befoie the Purge. ——Clyfters were ufed as in recent Cafes, where the Sick were low, or had much Pain of the Bowels (*n*), or complained of a Tenefmus.

In

(*n*) On the 21ft of *November*, 1759, *Hanah Meredith*, a middle-aged Woman, was admitted into *St. George*'s Hofpital for a Flux, which fhe had fix or feven Weeks ; fhe had no Fever, but complained much of Sicknefs and Gripes, and her Diforder had reduced her very low. During the two firft Weeks of her being in the Hofpital, fhe had two Vomits of Ipecacuana and four Dofes of Rhubarb ; and in the Intervals anodyne and aftringent Medicines, which made no Alteration in her Complaints. On the 2d of *December*, fhe told me, that two Years before fhe had had a Flux for above three Months, which had yielded to no Remedies till fhe was ordered repeated Clyfters, and that they had made a Cure in a fhort Time. I then

G 3 ordered

In fome old Dyfenteries, where the villous
Coat of the Inteſtines was much injured, I gave
the Cordial Draughts, with the Addition of Half
a Drachm of the *balfamum copaivi*, a Scruple
of the Extract of the Bark, and five Drops of

ordered an emollient Clyſter with a drachm of the *electuarium*
diafcordii, and a Scruple of the *tinctura thebaica*, to be given
twice a Day, which gave her almoſt immediate Relief; and
with the Affiſtance of fome Dofes of Rhubarb, and one or two
Vomits and occafional Opiates, removed her Diforder by the
Middle of *January*; though ſhe remained long weak, and troubled at Times with Gripes; but thefe Complaints were at laſt
got the better of by her taking fome Dofes of Rhubarb, and
drinking daily a Pint of Lime Water mixed with Half a Pint
of Milk.

Sarah Spencer, a middle-aged Woman, was admitted into *St.*
George's Hofpital the 9th of *November*, 1763, for a Flux, which
had continued for two Months, and reduced her very low. She
complained much of Sicknefs and Gripes; her Stools were
moſtly compofed of Mucus and Blood; her Pulfe was low, and
ſhe had no Fever, but a Whitenefs of the Tongue, and complained of Thirſt.—The firſt Day ſhe had a Vomit, and next
Day a Dofe of the purging faline oily Draught.—She was ordered to have an emollient Clyſter, with a Drachm of Diafcord,
and as much *tinctura thebaica*, given her every Evening;
and to have a Dofe of the faline oily Purge twice a Week, and
Opiates occafionally; by following this Courfe, and drinking
at Times the Chalk Julep, her Diforder was removed, and ſhe
was difcharged the Hofpital on the 30th of the fame Month.

the

the *tinctura thebaica*, three Times a Day. At
firſt, this Medicine ſeemed to promiſe much,
particularly in the Caſe of an old Invalid, *William Brookes*; who had been long ill of a Flux,
attended with Gripes and a Tenefmus. He
had uſed Variety of Remedies, without receiving any Benefit. For the firſt Fortnight,
after he began the Uſe of this Medicine, he
reſted well, and found great Relief; and ſeemed to be in a fair Way of doing well. But
the Diſorder being too far advanced before
he began to uſe it, he relapſed, and
died. On opening his Body, the inner Coats
of the Rectum and the lower Part of the Colon ſeemed to be reduced almoſt to a gelatinous Subſtance, and the other Coats were
black, approaching to a Gangrene —The ſame
Medicine gave Relief in other Caſes, but they
were too far advanced before it was adminiſtered. In theſe Caſes, when the villous Coat of
the Inteſtines was inflamed and very irritable,
the mucilaginous Medicines, the *pulvis e tra-
gacantha*, and ſuch others, were of Service;
and frequently Starch Clyſters and Anodynes

gave

gave Relief, when other Remedies had little Effect. Flower, boiled with Milk, and sweetened with Sugar, and given for Breakfast, as mentioned by Dr. *Pringle,* proved a good Palliative to some ; and the Starch and Gum Arabic, diffolved in Water, a good Drink to others. —Lime Water and Milk, drank to the Quantity of a Pint or a Quart a Day, was of use to a few, though it did not agree with all.

It was very common for Patients bad in the malignant Fever to be seized likewise with the Flux. Such Cases were always extremely dangerous ; and when the Fever was bad, we were often obliged to neglect the Flux, and only attend to the Fever.—When the Purging was violent, and appeared very early in the Fever, it often sunk the Patients, and soon carried them off: but where it was moderate, and did not appear till towards the Height or the Decline of the Fever, it often proved a Crisis to the Disorder.

When such Fluxes appeared early attended with sharp Pain of the Bowels, and Signs of Inflammation, if the Patient

was

was ftrong, we began the Cure with opening a Vein, which the Patient bore eafily,
and it gave Relief; but when the Symptoms were mild, without any acute Pain, the
Bleeding was omitted.—Commonly the Bowels
were loaded with corrupted Humours, when
this Symptom appeared; and, therefore, we
found it of Advantage to give a Dofe of the
Salts with Manna and Oil, or fome other gentle Purge, to carry them off; and in the Evening an Opiate to eafe the Pain and procure
the Patient Reft.

After this we gave the Mindereri Draughts
with Mithridate; and as foon as the Petechiæ appeared, or we obferved any Remiffions
in the Fever, the Patient took every four or
fix Hours, a Drachm of an Electuary, compofed of equal Parts of the *electuarium corticis*
and the *electuarium diafcordii* (*p*); or Half
a Drachm

(*p*) This Practice of giving the Cortex with Opiates in the
Dyfentery is not new; for Dr. R. *Morton*, in his Appendix to
his fecond Exercife on the Fevers, which appeared from 1658
to 1691, obferves, that after the Plague of 1666 had ceafed, a
Fever from a milder Poifon, attended with Gripes and Dyfentery, began to make its Appearance. As the common Methods

a Drachm of the Powder of the Bark, or a Scruple of the Extract, in the Mindereri Draughts, with four or five Drops of the *tinctura thebaica*; and we repeated the Opiate in the Evening, always proportioning the Quantity of it to the Effects of the former Dose, and the Violence of the Purging.

thods of Cure proved unsuccessful, and Dr. *Morton* observed Exacerbations and Remissions, he resolved to give the Bark mixed with Laudanum; and found it answer his Expectation. The first Patient to whom he gave it, was a man in *Long Lane*, who laboured under a Tertian Dysentery; upon observing a Remission, he ordered a Drachm of the Bark, mixed with a Grain of Opium, to be given every four Hours for six Times; and this removed both the Fever and Dysentery.—He says, he afterwards gave it, with equal Success, in the Quotidian Dysenteries, where he observed Exacerbations or Remissions; and he adds, that he does not doubt but that it will answer as well in Epidemical Diarrhœa's, and Camp Fevers attended with such Symptoms.

Dr. *Whytt* of *Edinburgh* has given with Success a strong Decoction of the Bark, mixed with the *confectio japonica* of the *Edinburgh* Dispensatory, in the bad State of the Dysentery, when the Mouth and alimentary Canal were threatened with Aphthæ, and even sometimes after they had appeared. And Dr. *Pringle* mentions his having given the Decoction of the Bark, wih Snake-Root and some Drops of Laudanum, in the Dysentery complicated with the malignant Fever. See *Note* *to Page* 245 *of his third Edition on the Diseases of the Army.*

On

On the fecond or third Day, we repeated the Purge; or, if the Patient was weak, ordered a Clyſter to be adminiſtered in its Place; in order to prevent the putrid Fluids and Excrements from being accumulated in the Bowels: —In other reſpeſts we treated it as when the Diſorder was not complicated with the malignant Fever.

This Method, though it did not ſucceed with all, yet it anſwered better than any other I tried;—and it ought to be remarked, that although it had ſuch a good Effeſt in Caſes attended with the malignant Fever, or where the Fever inclined to the intermittent Kind, it did not anſwer ſo well in other recent Caſes, but often made the Patient ſick.

In military Hoſpitals, Fluxes are liable to be complicated with other Diſorders, as well as with the malignant Fever; eſpecially with Coughs, and pleuritic and peripneumonic Symptoms, when the Weather begins to be cold, in *Oſtober* and *November.*—In ſuch Caſes, when the Patients were ſtrong, we were often obliged to bleed freely, to apply Bliſters, and in the

Beginning

Beginning treat the Diforder as inflammatory; having at the fame Time an Eye towards the Flux, in the other Medicines we prefcribed.

Patients, who have had the Flux long, are apt to have their Legs fwell at Nights; or to fwell all over as foon as the Flux has ftopped. Such oedematous or anafarcous Swellings, we treated nearly in the fame Manner as thofe which followed the petechial Fever; only that we durft not at firft be fo free with the Ufe of Purgatives; for as the Bowels remained weak and eafily irritated, fuch Medicines were apt to bring back the Flux; and therefore, in the Beginning, we were for the moft part obliged to attempt the Cure by Diuretics and Diaphoretics; and to be fparing of the Ufe of Purgatives, efpecially of thofe of the hydragogue Kind; though if the Swellings continued for fome Time after the Flux was gone off, and the Patients were ftrong, we then ventured to give Purges at proper Intervals:—And Blifters and Scarifications removed them in feveral Inftances both at *Paderborn* and *Ofnabruck.*

In

In *December*, 1761, we had a Cafe of this Kind where the *oxymel fcilliticum* was of remarkable Service. A Soldier, belonging to the Guards, after a Flux, fwelled all over, and made but a very fmall Quantity of Water. He took Medicines of different Sorts for fome Weeks, but received no Benefit till we gave him the Oxymel Mixture; after taking a few Dofes he made Water very freely, and in large Quantities, and the Swellings of his Body and Scrotum began immediately to fubfide; and by continuing its Ufe for a Fortnight, the Swellings entirely difappeared, and he recovered his Health and Strength.——The Oxymel, at the fame Time that it promoted a Flow of Urine, kept his Body gently open, but did not occafion any Return of the Flux.

At the Beginning of *January*, 1762, one *Carter*, a Soldier of the Eleventh Regiment of Foot, laboured under an univerfal Anafarca; which about two Months before had fucceeded a Flux. He made but very little Water, and that of a high red Colour. He took Variety

riety of Medicines, as Purges, Vomits, *Dover's*
Powder, lixivial and neutral Salts with Opiates,
Infufions of Horfe-Radifh, all without Effect;
till he was ordered fmall Dofes of Calomel,
three Grains Morning and Evening. After the
third Dofe he began to make Water freely ;
and by the 24th of *January* the Swellings were
all gone, and he was fhipped off for *England*
the 8th of *February*; having been difcharged
from his Regiment. The Ship, he went aboard
of, was detained in the River *Wefer* for above
fix Weeks, and the malignant Fever broke out
aboard the Tranfport : He took the Diftemper, and got well of it ; but towards the Decline was feized with a Return of the Flux,
which carried him off.

When thefe oedematous Swellings came after
the Purging was ftopt, if the Patient's Strength
was not much exhaufted, and he laboured under no other Diforder, he commonly got the
better of it :—But when the Strength was gone
before the Swellings appeared, the Diforder
often ended in a confirmed Dropfy, and at laft

in

in Death ; and when the Swellings were univerfal over the Body, while the Flux yet continued, it was a Sign of great Weaknefs, and they
did not furvive it long (*q*).

(*q*) Many other Medicines have been ufed for the Cure
of old Dyfenteries, ———— The *Coneffi Bark*, recommended
as a Specific in Diarrhœas, cured a Dyfentery which had
yielded nothing to a Variety of Medicines. *Edinburgh Medical
Effays, Vol.* III. *Art.* iv.—The *cortex eleutheriæ vel cafcarillæ* is
much recommended for the Cure of Dyfenteries in the *Memoir.
de L'Academie des Sciences a Paris* 1719, and is ftill in great Repute among the *Germans.*—The Decoction of the *femiruba* Bark
was found to have a good Effect in the Dyfentery, where the
Patient continued to void Blood with his Stools ; and when the
Stools were only liquid, without a Mixture of Blood, fome of
the Cafcarilla added to the Decoction encreafed its Efficacy.
See *Degnerus's* Treatife *de Dyfenteria, cap.* iii. *fect.* 55. Thefe
and many other Remedies have been tried in obftinate Dyfenteries.

From what I have obferved myfelf, and from the Accounts
of others, I am now convinced, that fuch Cafes as are not already too far gone, are moft likely to be cured,

1. By keeping the Patients on a low Diet, compofed principally of Milk, Sago, Rice, Salop, and fuch other Things as are
recommended by Dr. *Pringle*; allowing weak Breths, and a
fmall Quantity of white Meat, as they recover their Strength.
The common Drink to be Barley or Rice-Water, Toaft and
Water, *Briftol* Water, Almond Emulfion, and fuch like.—By
making them wear fome additional Cloathing, and guarding
carefully againft catching cold.—Errors of Diet and Expofure

to Cold being the moſt frequent Cauſes of Relapſes into this
Diſorder.

2. By giving from Time to Time a Doſe of ſome mild Purge;
ſuch as a little Manna and Salts ; a Solution of Manna in Almond Emulſion ; twenty or thirty Grains of Rhubarb, in a ſaline Draught, or ſuch like ; and occaſionally gentle Emetics.

3. By the Uſe of ſome of the mild Aſtringents and Corrobo-
rants.—The Bark, with Aſtringents and Opiates, agreeing beſt
with ſome —Decoctions of the Semiruba with others—Chalk in
Electuaries, or Juleps, with others—anodyne and aſtringent
Clyſters with others—while others receive more Benefit from
other Remedies—and ſeverals find themſelves better when they
uſe no Medicines of this Kind.

4. And by the occaſional Uſe of Opiates, and a free Air:
And by moderate Exerciſe on Horſeback, or in a Machine in
the convaleſcent State.

I ought not to omit mentioning, that I have ſeen ſome Caſes
where Evacuations had been uſed in the Beginning, which,
after they had continued for ſome Time, were cured by a
regular Diet of Broths, and white Meats; riding daily on Horſeback ; and drinking a generous good Claret Wine. However,
it ought to be remarked, that this Method only ſucceeded
where the Diſorder was mild, and its Violence had abated by
previous Evacuations.

O F

OF THE

CHOLERA MORBUS.

THE Cholera Morbus, or a fudden arid violent Vomiting and Purging, was very frequent in *July* and *Auguft* 1761 ; and feveral were attacked with it at *Munfter*.—It was attended with great Sicknefs, with Pain, and Inflation of the Abdomen, Thirft, and a fmall quick Pulfe : Some had it in a pretty violent Degree, but in general it was mild ; and although the Sicknefs, Vomiting, and Purging, continued, in one or two Cafes, for above a Day ; yet none of thofe died whom I faw.

This Diforder weakens the Patient much, in a fhort Space of Time ; and fometimes, when violent, kills in lefs than twenty-four Hours. It is always moft frequent in Summer and the

H   Beginning

Beginning of Autumn ; and is taken Notice of by *Hippocrates, Aretæus, Celfus*, and other antient Authors ; and is very accurately defcribed by many of them.—It is of the bilious Kind ; and the Cure principally depends upon the free Ufe of warm mild Liquors in the Beginning ; to dilute and blunt the Acrimony of the Bile, and other Fluids, and to promote their Difcharge ; and afterwards of gentle Cordials to fupport the Strength ; and warm Fomentations to allay the Pain when violent ; and mild Opiates to procure Reft ; and if the Sicknefs or Griping remains next Day after the Cholera is ftopt, to give a Dofe of Phyfic and an Opiate in the Evening.

An Officer, who had been wounded on the 15th of *July*, at the Battle of *Fillinghaufen*, began afterwards to live very freely, and was on the 4th of *Auguft* feized in the Night with the Cholera.—About ten o'Clock next Day I was fent for ; and found him in violent Agony, with fharp Pain in the Bowels, Reachings, and Strainings to Vomit, and Spafms and Cramps in the Bowels, Legs, and Arms.—He had large red

red Blotches on his Extremities, and no Pulfe was to be felt at the Wrift, and rather a Fluttering than a Beating at the Heart.—He had vomited and purged much in the Night before I faw him, but the Purging had begun to abate.—I immediately ordered him an emollient Clyfter, and a faline Draught, with the *confeſtio cardiaca,* and five Drops of liquid Laudanum; which, if he vomited up, was to be repeated foon after; if not, only once in four Hours: And he was directed to drink freely of weak Chicken Broth, warm.—Two Hours afterwards we found him in the fame Situation; ftill no Pulfe to be felt, which prevented us from bleeding him; and the violent Pain of the Stomach and Bowels, and the Cramps, continued. We then ordered Flannels, dipped in a warm emollient Decoction, to be kept conftantly applied to his Belly, dipping them in the warm Decoction as foon as they began to grow cool; his Clyfter to be repeated with the Addition of a Drachm of the *electuarium e baccis lauri,* and Half a Drachm of the *tinctura thebaica;* a Scruple of Caftor, and Half a

Drachm

Drachm of Spirit of Lavender, to be added to each of his Draughts; and a Blifter to be prepared, in cafe thefe Medicines gave no Relief. —Soon after, beginning to ufe the Fomentations, the Cramps and Pains began to abate; about four o'Clock in the Afternoon we could perceive a Fluttering of the Pulfe at the Wrift, and all the Pains and Cramps were much eafier; fo that there was no occafion for the Blifter.—Next Morning he was very eafy, but low, and inclined to be fick; for which his Cordial Draughts were repeated every fix Hours.—The third Day, as he complained cf a little Griping in the Bowels, we ordered him a Dofe of Tincture of Rhubarb, and an Opiate in the Evening, which entirely removed thefe Complaints, and he was abroad and well next Day.

One Soldier, who had a good deal of Fever, and complained of acute Pain in the Bowels, along with the Vomiting and Purging, was blooded; and drank freely of warm Barley-Water while the Vomiting continued.——After throwing up a Quantity of green bilious Mat-

ter,

ter, the Vomiting ceafed ; and the Gripes and Purging became lefs violent.—In an Hour after, being able to retain fome very weak Broth in his Stomach, he drank plentifully of it through the Day ; and the Purging being abated towards Night, he took an anodyne Draught ; and next Day, having ftill a little Sicknefs remaining, had a Dofe of Phyfic and an Opiate at Night, which removed all his Complaints.

The Reft, who were attacked with the Cholera at *Munfter*, were treated much in the fame Way ; only as they had not fuch acute Pain and Fever as this Man, it was thought unneceffary to bleed them.

The Antients (*r*) recommended drinking freely of warm Water in the Beginning, and the Ufe of both cold and hot Fomentations of the Stomach and Belly ;—and in the low State, the Ufe of Wine, mixed with Water, and Polenta (*s*) ; and to apply Rue, with Vinegar, and

(*r*) See *Aretæus*, Lib. ii. Cap. 4. and *Celfus*, Lib. iv. Cap. 11.

(*s*) The Polenta feems to have been nothing but toafted Barley Meal. See *Plinii Hift. Natural.* Lib. xxii. Cap. 25.

H 3   other

other ftrong fmelling Things, to the Noftrils; befides Variety of other Remedies. —When Convulfions happen, *Celfus* (*t*) advifes to anoint the Belly with warm Oil ; and if that does not remove them, to apply Cupping-Glaffes or Muftard to the Stomach ; and, after fleeping, to abftain the fecond Day from Drink ; and the third, to go into the Bath ; and if any thing of a Fever remains after the Cholera is fuppreffed, to give a Purge.

Dr. *Sydenham* (*u*) trufts principally to drinking freely of Chicken Broth, and throwing up Clyfters of the fame, and afterwards giving Opiates.

Dr. *Ayton Douglas*, in the fixth Volume of the *Edinburgh* Medical Effays (*w*), recommends a Decoction of Oat Bread, baked without Leaven or Yeft, and carefully toafted as brown as Coffee, but not burnt; as a Remedy very grateful to the Stomach, and ufeful in ftopping the Vomiting, and fometimes the Purging too: And he relates feveral Cafes

(*t*) *Celfus loco citato.*
(*u*) *Proceffus integ. de Cholera.*
(*w*) Art. 65.

where

where it had a good Effect. After the Vomit-
ing was ftopped, he added the Ufe of mild
Opiates ; and, where the Patient was low,
Wine and other Cordials.

H 4   O F

OF THE

INFLAMMATORY FEVER,

O N the Return of the Troops from the Winter Expedition into the Country of *Heſſe*, in the Year 1761, we had ſeveral Men ſeized with Inflammatory Fevers without any topical Inflammation ; and at the Opening of each Campaign had always Numbers ſent to the Hoſpitals ill of this Diſorder. Towards the End of the Campaigns, and throughout the Winter, many were ſeized with Inflammatory Fevers ; but theſe were moſtly complicated, with pleuritic, or peripneumonic Symptoms, or other topical Inflammations, or with rheumatic Complaints.

In the Inflammatory Fever, the Sick were ſeized at firſt with cold and hot Fits, ſucceeded

by

by Pain in the Head and all over the Body.
The Pulfe was ftrong and quick, and the Blood
fizy; attended with other Appearances commonly obferved in fuch Fevers.

As the Summer advanced, this Fever was
often accompanied with bilious Symptoms,
with Sicknefs, and vomiting of bilious Matter,
and very frequently with a Purging: Towards
the End of Summer it ceafed, and was fucceeded by the bilious remittent Fever.—And
it was no uncommon Thing to fee thofe Fevers, which originally were entirely of an inflammatory Nature, after the Sick had been
fome Days in a crowded Hofpital, partake a
good deal of the Nature of the Malignant Fever, or be changed entirely into it.

We treated thefe Fevers in the common
antiphlogiftic Method.—We blooded freely
in the Beginning; gave the faline Draughts
with Nitre and other cooling Medicines; and
made the Patients drink plentifully of fmall
Liquors:—And when they were inclined to
be coftive, gave mild Purges, or emollient
laxative Clyfters. We afterwards applied Blif-

ters;

ters; and if the Pulfe began to fink, gave Cordials, Wine, and other Remedies commonly employed in fuch Cafes;—and towards the Decline of the Fever endeavoured to promote fuch Evacuations as were pointed out by Nature, and likely to prove critical.

When the Cafe was complicated with bilious Symptoms in the Beginning, we were obliged to have particular Regard to the firft Paffages. If the Patient complained much of Sicknefs, we gave a gentle Vomit in the Evening, after bleeding; and a Purge next Day, to carry off any bilious or corrupted Humours that might be lodged in the Stomach or Inteftines; and we found that thefe Evacuations gave Relief, and generally mitigated all the Symptoms.

If at any Time during the Fever a Loofenefs came on, efpecially when attended with Gripes, we gave a Dofe of fome gentle Phyfic, which made a free Evacuation; and an Opiate in the Evening after its Operation; and afterwards we found it anfwer better to attempt rather to moderate, than wholly ftop the Purging

ing by ſtrong Aſtringents, and Opiates; unleſs where the Evacuation by Stool was ſo great as to be in Danger of ſinking the Patient.

The *pulvis antimonialis*, compoſed of ten Parts of the *pulvis e chelis*, and one Part of the Tartar emetic, given in ſmall Doſes, was ſerviceable in many of theſe Fevers, after free Evacuations had been made.

Two Patients, one a Soldier of the Twentieth Regiment, the other a *German* Waggoner, were taken ill of this Fever about the 25th of *December*, 1762 : They were both blooded freely, and had a Doſe of Phyſic in the Beginning; and the ſaline Draughts with Nitre and other cooling Remedies; and had Bliſters applied without producing any conſiderable Change in their Diſorder.—On the 5th of *January*, 1763, they both complained much of Thirſt, and were inclined to be coſtive ; their Tongues were parched, their Pulſes quick and ſmall, and their Skins dry ; they were reſtleſs at Nights, and the Soldier had a ſlight Delirium.—I ordered each of them four Grains of the *pulvis antimonialis* every four Hours.

6th.

6th. Next Day the Soldier told me, he had had four loose Stools ; his Senses were much clearer, the Pulse calmer and flower, and he said he found himself lighter and easier, and less feverish, than he had been since he was first taken ill. The Medicine was continued, with the Addition of an anodyne Draught at Night.—7th. I found him in a fine breathing Sweat, and he told me he had slept well in the Night: p.——8th. The Sweat continued till this Morning, and on going off his Urine let fall a copious white Sediment, and left him free from the Fever ; after which he mended daily.

The Waggoner, after taking the third Dose of the Powders, had a warm Moisture upon the Skin.—On the 6th was cooler and without much Fever, and had had one Stool.—7th. The warm Moisture ended in a profuse Sweat, which carried off the Fever, and he continued to recover daily.

O F

OF THE

A N G I N A ;

O R,

S O R E T H R O A T.

M ANY of the Soldiers during the Campaign were feized with Inflammations
of the Throat, efpecially when the Nights were
cold and moift after warm Days ; and when
they did Duty in cold wet Nights in the Winter
Seafon.—All of them I faw in *Germany* were
of the inflammatory Kind ; I did not obferve
any that were malignant.

They were treated in the antiphlogiftic
Method.—The Patients were blooded liberally

in

in the Beginning—took the cooling nitrous and faline Medicines——gentle Diaphoretics and Purgatives——and ufed frequent Gargarifms.

Sometimes a Flannel rubbed with campho-rated Oil, or the *linimentum volatile*, and ap-plied round the Neck, was of Service.——And frequently after bleeding fufficiently, where the Breathing or Swallowing was difficult, the Ap-plication of a large Blifter to the Neck gave fpeedy Relief.

O F

OF THE

PLEURISY.

THE Pleurify, or an acute Inflammation of the Side, was moſt frequent among the Soldiers towards the latter End of the Campaigns; though ſome were attacked with it at all Times of the Year, from doing Duty in all Sorts of Weather.

We followed the antiphlogiſtic Method of Cure; and ordered plentiful Bleeding in the Beginning, till the Violence of the Pain began to abate, or the Patient grew faint;—and the Side to be fomented with Flannels dipped in warm emollient Decoctions, and afterwards rubbed with volatile Liniments: At the ſame Time the Patient drank freely of warm diluting

ing Liquors, as Barley Water, the pectoral Decoction, and such like; and took the saline
and other cooling Medicines, mixed occa-
sionally with Sperma Ceti, or some other soft
Pectorals, if there was a tickling Cough.——
When the Patient was costive, we gave a Dose
of Salts, or some other mild Physic, or laxative Clysters.

If the Pain continued very acute, we repeated the Bleeding as often as Necessity seemed to require, and the Pulse could bear; and
immediately after the second Bleeding ordered
a large Blister to be applied to the Part affected.

Physicians formerly used to forbid Bleeding
·after the fourth Day, if it had been omitted so
long; but when no Symptoms of Suppuration
had already appeared, on whatever Day of the
Disorder it happened, I ordered plentiful Bleeding, the same as in recent Cases; and never
found any Disadvantage, but often great Service from this Practice.

When the Sharpness of the Pain was gone,
and the Pulse became soft, very often a dull

' Pain

Pain remained for fome Time in the Part.———
In fome Cafes a brifk Purge removed it;—in
others, cupping above the Part, and afterwards
rubbing it with the volatile Liniments, did Service;—in others, gentle Opiates at Night, efpecially where there was a tickling Cough;—
and in one or two Cafes, this Pain did not go
away, till the Patient was ordered to drink every
Day for fome Time, a Quart of the Decoction
of Sarfaparilla with the antimonial Wine.

In the Courfe of this Diforder, if a kindly
Moifture broke out on the Skin, which gave
Relief, this was encouraged by the Ufe of mild
warm Liquors; or if the Patient began to fpit
up a vifcid or yellowifh Mucus, we endeavoured to keep up the Expectoration by the Ufe of
mild Pectorals; and if a Purging came on, we
were careful not to check it too foon, unlefs it
was fo violent as to be in Danger of finking the
Patient.

When an Inflammation of the Side came to
Suppuration, which happened in one or two
Cafes at *Ofnabruck*, in *May* 1761; as foon as a
Fluctuation of Matter was to be felt, an Incifion

I   was

was made in the Part, and the Matter diſcharged; after which the Sore healed kindly, and the Patients recovered (*a*). I am perſuaded, was this Operation oftener performed, many would recover who die conſumptive.

(*a*) Dr. *Mead* adviſes, where the Lungs and Pleura grow together, and an Abſceſs forms, to open it with Cauſtic; and afterwards to keep the Ulcer open during the Patient's Life: For he ſays, he has often ſeen, where ſuch Sores were healed up, that the Patient died ſoon after by an Efflux of Matter upon the Breaſt. *Monita Medica,* Cap. i. Sect. 7.

O F

PERIPNEUMONY.

THE Soldiers were subject at all Times to the Peripneumony, or Inflammation of the Lungs, from doing Duty in cold wet Weather, and from their irregular Way of living; but more particularly towards the End of the Campaigns, and in Winter.

This Diforder was much more dangerous and fatal than the Pleurify, efpecially when neglected in the Beginning; for then Bleeding had feldom any Effect; the Difficulty of Breathing encreafed, the Patient was feized with an Orthopnea, and fuch an Anxiety and Senfe of Suffocation, that he could not fleep; and the Pulfe funk; and in thefe Cafes Death only afforded Relief. This we experienced in many

I 2   Men

Men who had lain neglected in Quarters, for two, three, four, or five Days, before they were brought to the Hofpital.

In moft of the Bodies of thofe who died of this Diforder, and were opened after Death; we found the Lungs violently inflamed, with livid or gangrenous Spots on their Surface; and more or lefs of a watery Serum extravafated into the Cavity of the Cheft.

Three had Suppurations in the Lungs. In one, who had lain fick in Quarters for ten Days or upwards, before he was fent to the Hofpital, the right Cavity of the Thorax was found full of a watery Serum; and the Lobes of the Lungs on the fame Side almoft entirely wafted; and what remained feemed as it were compofed of thickened Membranes, refembling thofe form-ed by the coagulable Lymph, or what is called by fome (though improperly) the fibrous Part of the Blood. The Lobes in the left Side feemed to be in a found State, or at moft but flightly inflamed. From the right Lobes of the Lungs being fo much wafted, I fufpected that the Patient had probably laboured long under

under fome Diforder of the Breaſt; but I could not from Enquiry obtain any Information in this Particular; nor did he ever mention ſuch a Thing during the few Days he lived after being brought into the Hoſpital; he ſaid, he had only been ill for eight or ten Days before; but Soldiers afflicted with chronic Diſtempers, when they are ſeized with violent Symptoms, or acute Diſeaſes, are apt to reckon the Beginning of their Diforder, only from the Time they are taken ill in a violent Manner; and never to take any Notice of their former Complaints.

Another Soldier, about the Middle of *February*, 1762, remained in Quarters five Days after being taken ill with a Pain of the Breaſt, and a Difficulty of Breathing; the ſixth Day he was brought to the Hoſpital in the Morning, and I ſaw him about eleven o'Clock; he then had all the Symptoms of the true Peripneumony, attended with a ſtrong hard Pulſe. He was immediately blooded as freely as his Pulſe would bear, had Bliſters applied, and other Remedies uſed; notwithſtanding which,

I 3

on

on the eighth Day from that Time, he began to throw up a purulent Matter in great Quantity, attended with a conftant hectic Heat, and Fever; which funk him fo faft, that he died the tenth Day, after he firft began to expectorate.

On the 2d of *March*, a Soldier, of the Fifty-firft Regiment of Foot, was brought to the Hofpital, with a violent Pain in the left Side, and a great Difficulty of Breathing. Upon examining him, he told me, that about two Years before he had had a violent Stitch in his left Side, towards the lower Part of the Thorax; that ever fince he had been fubject to a Difficulty of Breathing; and at Times to a Pain in the Side; but that he had only been feized with the violent Pain and Difficulty of Breathing he then complained of, about five Days before, occafioned by catching Cold, on being billeted in a low, cold, and damp Houfe.—His Pulfe was quick, the Pain of his Side and Difficulty of Breathing fo great, that he could not fleep, nor lie down, but was obliged to fit conftantly in an erect Pofture; his Tongue was

white

white and furred, and he had had no Stools for three Days : He was ordered to be blooded immediately; and to take a Dose of Salts; and his Side to be rubbed with the *linimentum volatile*. 3d. His Breathing and Pain of the Side were easier; he had slept a little in the Night, and could lie on his right side, but not on his left. He was ordered the Squill Mixture. 4th. His Breathing was worse ; he was blooded a second Time ; had a large Blister applied to his Side, and was ordered to continue the Use of the Squill Mixture. On the 5th, 6th, and 7th, he seemed easier, though the Breathing was still much affected, and his Pulse quick and low, attended with a hectic Heat. On the 8th, he told me that his left Side was swelled : On examining, I observed a Fullness in that Side of the Thorax ; and on pressing with my Fingers between the Ribs, I thought I felt an obscure Fluctuation of a deep-seated Fluid. From these Appearances, and the History of the Case, I judged that there was a Collection of some Fluid within the Cavity of the Chest ;

and

and that the only Means left to give Relief, was to make an Opening into the Cavity, and fo evacuate the Fluid. I therefore propofed to him the Operation of the Empyema, to be performed immediately ; which he feveral Times obftinately refufed to fubmit to : He allowed a Seton to be put in his Side, but that did not anfwer the End propofed : He languifhed fix Days longer ; and died the 14th of *March.* Next Day an Opening was made in the Thorax, in the Part where the Operation was propofed to have been performed ; as foon as the Pleura was cut through, fome Quarts of Water rufhed out. We then opened the Thorax, and found ftill fome Water in the left Cavity. The Pericardium was thickened, and flightly inflamed, and adhered to the Diaphragm ; which was likewife a little thickened and inflamed in the adhering Part ; the Lungs on that Side were much compreffed, and contracted by the Preffure of the Water ; but on being inflated and cut, feemed in a found State, except that they were flightly inflamed. The

Lungs

Lungs of the left Side adhered every-where firmly to the Thorax, but feemed otherwife found; having no Tubercles, Suppuration, or other Diforder, that we could obferve in cutting them. The Heart and Blood Veffels were found, and no other polypous Concretions were obferved within their Cavities, but fuch as we find in moft dead Bodies; which feem to be formed of the coagulable Lymph in *articulo mortis.* The Vifcera of the Abdomen were in a found State.

We treated the Peripneumony nearly as the Pleurify. We bled freely in the Beginning, till the Breathing became eafier, or the Pulfe began to fink ; taking Care not to be deceived by a low oppreffive Pulfe, which generally rofe upon Bleeding. We applied large Blifters; gave the mild Pectorals freely, and plenty of warm diluting Liquors, Barley Water, the pectoral Decoction, and fuch like ; which afforded more Relief than any other Medicines. We gave too faline Purges, and laxative Clyfters occafionally ; and in fome Cafes ordered the

Steams

Steams of warm emollient Decoctions with Vinegar to be drawn into the Lungs.

By this Treatment moft of them, who applied early for Relief, got the better of the Diforder.

When the Expectoration began, the Patient continued the free Ufe of the mild Pectorals, and diluting Liquors ; and no Medicines were given that might in the leaft tend to ftop it ; other Evacuations were omitted, unlefs where the Pain of the Breaft, or the Difficulty of Breathing increafed ; in which Cafe, if the Pulfe kept up, I ordered a Vein to be opened, and a fuitable Quantity of Blood to be taken away ; no other Remedy affording any Relief, till this Evacuation was made. Where the Patient was coftive, we frequently ordered laxative Clyfters, or a mild Purge, and found them beneficial : But where no fuch Symptoms occurred, it was beft, for the moft part, to omit all Evacuations of this Kind, after a free Expectoration had begun, and to truft to it for carrying off the Diforder.

In

In fome Cafes, where the Expectoration ftopt fuddenly after bleeding, we gave with Advantage a gentle Vomit, as recommended by Dr. *Huxham* (*a*).

(*a*) Some late Authors feem to look upon the *Pleurify* and *Peripneumony* as the fame Diforder: However, though it be true, that when the *Pleura* is inflamed, the Surface of the contiguous Lungs is generally in the fame State ; and that, when the *Lungs* are inflamed, the Pleura is often affected ; yet as I have frequently feen the true Peripneumony without that fharp Pain of the Side which characterizes the Pleurify; and upon opening the Bodies of People who have died of the Peripneumony, have found the Lungs violently inflamed and livid, and fo filled with Blood as to fink in Water, without the Pleura being much difeafed ; and upon opening the Thorax of others who died of the Pleurify, have found the intercoftal Mufcles and Pleura violently inflamed with livid Spots, and only a fmall Portion of the Surface of the contiguous Lungs affected ; I cannot help ftill looking upon them as diftinct Diforders ; though they require nearly the fame Treatment, and are often complicated together.

O F

OF THE

Cough and Consumption.

COUGHS were very frequent during the Winter, and when the Weather was wet and cold. They were often accompanied with Pains of the Breaſt; and, when neglected, Obſtructions, Tubercles, and Suppurations, were apt to form in the Lungs, and the Diſeaſe to end in a Conſumption, or *Phthiſis Pulmonalis.*

When Coughs were ſlight, guarding againſt further Cold, and the Uſe of mild Pectorals and warm Drinks, removed them. But when the Patient complained of a Pain and Tightneſs about the Breaſt, it was always neceſſary to take away more or leſs Blood; and after Bleeding to give ſome of the mild Pectorals, ſuch as

the

the Sperma Ceti or oily Mixtures; and, if a
Fever attended, to join the Ufe of Nitre, or of
the faline or mindereri Draughts; and, if a
tickling Cough was troublefome, to give frequently a Tea Spoonful of the oily Linctus, acidulated either with the Spirit of Vitriol, or the
oxymel fcilliticum. The mild Diaphoretics,
fuch as the mindereri Draughts, given along
with warm Drinks, to promote a free Perfpiration, or Sweat, were ufed with Advantage;
when the Patients kept in Bed, and lay in
Wards which had Stoves in them.

If the Cough and Pain of the Breaft were
not relieved by thefe Means, the Patient was
bled a fecond Time, and a Blifter applied to the
Side immediately after; which often removed
moft of the Complaints. When it did not,
we gave the pectoral Decoction for common
Drink; and if there was a Shortnefs or Difficulty of Breathing, the fquill Mixture, or *lac
ammoniacum*, with Oxymel; and occafionally
gentle Purges: And if at any Time of the
Diforder the Tightnefs and Pain of the Breaft
returned

returned violent, we took away fome Blood, no other Remedy affording Relief.

When there was little or no Fever, and a thin Rheum kept up a tickling Cough, nothing had a better Effect than to add fome Drops of the *tinctura thebaica*, or fome of the *elixir paregoricum*, to the oleagenous or fquill Mixtures; or to give an Opiate Draught or Pill at Bed-Time, which eafed the Cough, and procured the Patient Reft.

At all Times it was neceffary, when the Cough was violent, attended with Pains of the Breaft, to keep the Patients on low Diet; and in as free and pure Air as the Nature of the Hofpitals would admit of; for we often found that thofe Men who had laboured long under obftinate Coughs, which threatened Confumptions in fmall crowded Wards, recovered furprifingly on being removed to a freer Air; of which we had a remarkable Inftance in the Hofpital at *Bremen*, in *January* 1762; upon removing fome Men, afflicted with very bad Coughs, out of fmall Wards, which were damp, into one large one, which was dry and airy.

When

When the Weather was good, we made the Patients walk out a little in the Day-Time; for we ob'erved, that remaining always in the Hofpital, and breathing nothing but a foul Air, helped to encreafe the Diforder.—When we knew the Men to be fober, and not apt to commit Irregularities, we ufed to procure them good Billets, and make them come daily to the Hofpital for their Medicines.

Equal Parts of Lime-Water and Milk, drank to the Quantity of a Quart a Day, was of Ufe to fome; and the *infufum amarum*, and other gentle Bitters, taken to the Quantity of an Ounce or two, Morning and Evening, to others (*a*).

(*a*) Affes Milk, and *Briftol* and *Seltzer* Waters, which are found fo ferviceable in pulmonic Diforders, could not be had in the military Hofpitals; and riding on Horfeback was too expenfive a Remedy for a Soldier.

In chronic Cafes, where we fufpeft Obftruftions and Tubercles to be formed in the Lungs, which have not already come to Suppuration, Dr. *Ruffel* recommends the Ufe of Sea Water for refolving them; but we were at too great a Diftance from the Sea to try this Remedy. See his *Treatife on Sea Water*, Page 17.

A

A Decoction of the Cortex removed fome Coughs which had continued for a confiderable Time. In one or two of thefe Cafes, flight hectic Symptoms had already appeared (*b*). However, for the moft part, where-ever Obftructions of the Lungs were confirmed, or there were evident hectic Symptoms without

(*b*) *Mary Shepperd*, a Woman twenty-fix Years of Age, was admitted into *St. George*'s Hofpital the 6th of *June*, 1759, for a Cough; attended with a conftant hectic Fever and Night Sweats, which had begun in the Month of *April*, after the Meafles. She complained likewife of having the *fluor albus*, and fhe had been blooded more than once before fhe came to the Hofpital.—I at firft gave her fome of the mild Pectorals; and a Solution of White Vitriol in Water, *utenda pro inject. uterina*. After a Week, finding no Alteration in her Complaints, I advifed her to become an Out-patient; and to go down to her Friends in the Country, to live upon a Milk Diet; to take gentle Exercife, and continue the Ufe of her Medicines; which fhe did, but without any Alteration in her Diforder, till the 6th of *July*, when I ordered her to take thrice a Day two Ounces of the Decoction of the Cortex, along with a faline Draught. Immediately, on beginning to ufe this Medicine, her Diforder began to take a favourable Turn; her Fever and Night Sweats left her, her Cough became eafier, and fhe recovered Health and Strength daily. She came to the Hofpital the 15th of *Auguft*, feemingly in good Health, to return Thanks for her Cure.

a free

a free Difcharge of purulent Matter, the Bark ·
did no Service; but rather heated and increafed
the Fever, and made the Sick more reftlefs and
uneafy.—It was of moft Ufe where there
feemed to be no confirmed Obftruĉtions, but
the Veffels much relaxed; which we judged
to be the Cafe from the Patients having no
fixed Pain, nor the Breathing much affeĉted.
If the Sick were plethoric, or in the leaft feverifh, we ordered a little Blood to be taken
away, before we began the Ufe of this Medicine.

In fimilar Cafes, I have fometimes obferved
good Effeĉts from the Ufe of the Balfam *Co-
paivy*, or *Peru*; given either in Juleps or made
up into an Eleĉtuary, as in the *eleĉtuarium e
fpermate ceti cum balfamo*; but in whatever
Form they were given, if there were confirmed Obftruĉtions of the Lungs, they rather
heated and inflamed, than did any real Service.

When Coughs continued long, attended
with Pain in the Side, Difficulty of Breathing,
and Heĉtic Fever and Night Sweats, we always

had

had Reafon to fufpect, that the Diforder would terminate in a confirmed Confumption. When this was threatened, we found, that the principal Thing to be done, was to keep the Patients cool; and to endeavour to allay the hectic Heat and Fever; and to retard, as much as poffible, the Progrefs of the Diforder. When the Cafe was recent, we were fometimes fo lucky as to make a Cure; but after it was confirmed, it for the moft part ended fatally.

We kept the Patients upon a low Diet; and where-ever Milk was to be got eafily, we allowed them a Pint a Day (c); which was either mixed with Water and given for Drink, or they took it to Breakfaft or Supper.—Their common Drink was either Barley Water or the pectoral Decoction; which was occafionally acidulated with a few Drops of Spirit of

(c) In private Practice, at this Stage of the Diforder, the Ufe of Affes Milk, and drinking the *Briftol* Water at the *Briftol* Wells, and riding on Horfeback daily, are juftly ranked amongft the moft efficacious Remedies; and going into the more fouthern Climates, as the South of *France, Portugal*, or *Italy*, where the Air is warmer, more conftant, and dry, than in *England*, has often been found to produce good Effects.

Vitriol;

Vitriol; and we gave at the fame Time the cooling Medicines, fuch as Nitre, the faline or mindereri Draughts, mixed at Times with Sperma Ceti, or fome other of the mild Pecto-rals.

The opening a Vein, and taking away from four to eight Ounces of Blood (*d*), whenever the Pain of the Breaft was troublefome, or the Patient was hot and reftlefs at Nights from the Hectic Fever, gave the greateft Relief of any Thing we tried; and thefe repeated fmall Bleedings were fo far from wafting the Pa-tient's Strength, that they rather feemed to pre-vent its being exhaufted fo faft as otherwife it would have been, by allaying the Force of the Hectic Fever.

At this Stage of the Diforder, we put in Se-tons, or ordered Iffues, to ferve as a Drain to carry off the Matter, and found them of Ad-vantage in fome Cafes. When the Patients

(*d*) This Practice has been ftrongly recommended by Dr. *Mead*, in his *Monita Medica*, Sect. x. and by an anonymous Author in the *Edinburgh Medical Effays*, Vol. IV. Art. 28. and Dr. *Mead* fays, when Things have not been quite defperate, he has feen good Succefs from it.

complained

complained of any fixed Pain, we always made
the Iſſues as near the Part affected as poſſible (*e*). On the 5th of *May*, 1762, a Man,
belonging to the Eighty-eighth Regiment of
Foot, was ſent to the Hoſpital at *Bremen* for
an Hæmoptoe, attended with a conſtant hectic
Heat and Fever.—After being blooded, and
uſing the cooling Remedies without Succeſs,
he had four Pea Iſſues made in his Back; and
had a ſlight Decoction of the Cortex, acidulated

(*c*) In *June*, 1748, a Servant Girl came to aſk my Advice for
a Cough, attended with a conſtant Hectic Fever and Night
Sweats, which had begun ſome Months before, on catching
Cold. The Matter ſhe ſpit up was yellow, and had the Ap-
pearance of Pus; and ſhe complained of a Pain in the left Side
of the Thorax. I ordered her the ſaline Mixture with Sperma
Ceti to be taken thrice a Day, to loſe a little Blood, to drink
an Infuſion of Linſeed ſweetened with Honey, and to have a
Seton put in her Side at the Part where ſhe complained of
Pain; adviſing her to go home to her Father, who was a Far-
mer in the Country, and to live upon a Milk and Vegetable
Diet, and ride on Horſeback whenever ſhe could conveniently.
She ſeemed ſo far gone in a Conſumption, that I ſcarce expected to ſee her again; but, in the Month of *December*, ſhe
came to return me Thanks for her Cure, ſeeming then to be in
good Health. She told me, that, as ſoon as the Seton began to
diſcharge freely, ſhe found Relief; and mended afterwards
daily, by following the Directions I had given her.

with

with Spirit of Vitriol. As foon as the Iffues began to difcharge freely, the hectic Heat, Fever, and Spitting of Blood, diminifhed daily; and he recovered his Health and Strength in a fhort Time. However, it ought to be obferved, that although thefe Drains are fometimes efficacious, yet, when the Difeafe is far advanced, the Mifchief is generally too deep rooted for them to be of any Service.

The Bark, and natural Balfams, for the moft part were prejudicial, and encreafed the Hectic Heat and Fever; except in one or two Cafes, where the Diforder feemed to depend on a Vomica of the Lungs, and the Patient coughed up the Matter freely.—In one Cafe they were of confiderable Service; the Patient was very low, and had the Night Sweats, but coughed up the Matter freely : On ufing the Decoction of the Bark, and the *electuarium e fpermate ceti cum balfamo*, the Matter expectorated became thicker, and of a more balmy Confiftence, without any Increafe of Heat or Fever; after which the Symptoms became gradually milder, and the Patient recovered.

K 3　　　　　　　　　　　　In

In the Courfe of this Diforder the Patients often became very hot and reftlefs, and were troubled with Gripes, fucceeded by a Purging: Thefe Symptoms were moft readily removed by a Dofe of Rhubarb, or of fome other mild Purge ; for they generally proceeded from corrupted Humours lodged in the Inteftines. In the Evening, after the Operation of the Purge, we gave an Opiate to procure the Patient Reft.—When the firft Dofe of Phyfic did not ftop the Purging, we repeated the Opiates at Nights, and in a Day or two gave another Purge ; and if there was much Sicknefs, or Load at the Stomach, gave likewife a gentle Emetic.

If the Purging ftill continued, we were obliged to join the Ufe of Aftringents along with the Opiates. In fome Cafes, I found good Effects from equal Parts of Milk and Water boiled with Rofe Leaves, Pomegranate Bark, Balauftine Flowers, and Cinnamon, as recommended by Dr. *Mead* in his *Monita Medica* (*f*) ; it ferved

(*f*) Sect. x, *de Febrib. lentis five Hecticis.*

both

both for Food and Medicine.—When Opiates and Aftringents were given to ftop the Purging at its firft Appearance, before the Bowels were emptied, they always did Mifchief; and increafed the Heat and Fever: And although they ftopt the Purging for a few Hours, it always broke out with greater Violence afterwards.

When the Sick were attacked with a Shortnefs and Difficulty of Breathing, which was not relieved by Evacuations, and the Ufe of cooling Medicines, and Pectorals, and Blifters, nothing gave fo much Eafe, or had fuch a good Effect, as a gentle Vomit; for it often removed the immediate Oppreffion from the Breaft, and helped to pump up the Matter from the Lungs.

In the advanced State of the Confumption, the Cough was always very troublefome; and the Sick found no Relief but from Opiate Medicines, which, in fuch Cafes, cannot be expected to do more than give a little prefent Eafe.—As they were apt to obftruct the free Expectoration, we generally mixed them with

K 4   fome

fome *oxymel fcilliticum*, or *tinctura fœtida*, which took off a good deal of their fuffocating Quality.

Dr. *Barry* (*g*) advifes for the Cure of a Confumption, to make an Incifion or Aperture into the Side ; where-ever there is a fixed Pain attended with a Weight, a Hectic Fever, and other Symptoms of an evident Suppuration : He fays the Pleura is thickened, and the Lungs adhere at the Part where they are exulcerated ; and that by the Operation the Pus may be eva-cuated, and a Cure made ; and he gives feve-ral Inftances of the Succefs of the Operation, when performed in Time.

(*g*) *Treatife on the Digeftions,* p. 410.

O F

OF THE

Epidemical CATARRHAL FEVER

Of A P R I L, 1762 ;

C A L L E D,

THE INFLUENZA.

AFTER a very cold fevere Winter at
Bremen, the Weather, from being very
cold, became of a fudden extremely hot, about
the 10th of *April*. In a few Days after, many
People were feized with a violent Catarrhal
Diforder. It often began with fuch a Cold
and Shivering, that many imagined at firft that
they were going to have Agues ; but foon after
they were attacked with a Cough, and a Difficulty

culty of Breathing, and Pain of the Breaft, with a Head-Ach, and Pains all over the Body, efpecially in the Limbs.—The firft Nights they commonly had profufe Sweats.—In feveral, it had the Appearance of a remitting Fever, for the two or three firft Days.—Many had a flight Inflammation of the Throat, and a Hoarfenefs. In all it was attended with an acute Fever in the Beginning, and the Urine was of a high Colour ; and when the Diforder had put on the Appearance of a Remittent Fever in the Beginning, it dropt a Sediment towards Morning after the fecond Day ; and did the fame in all, when the Diforder was going off.—Some had a Purging, but the greater Number were rather inclined to be coftive.—The Cough in many was very violent ; and the Patients, after each Fit of Coughing, had Reachings, or Strainings to vomit, exactly refembling thofe which come after violent Fits of the Hooping Cough.—At firft the Patients fpit up only a little Phlegm ; but in the Decline of the Diforder, they expectorated freely.—The violent Cough and Feverifhnefs generally continued for four, five,

or

or fix Days ; with others it continued longer ; and fome had a Cough for two or three Weeks after the Fever left them.

This Catarrhal Fever feized moft of the People of the Town of *Bremen*; and there were very few of the *Britifh* who efcaped it ; at the fame Time, it was epidemical in moft Countries in *Europe*.

We treated it entirely as an inflammatory Diforder, and none died who applied early for Relief.—Moft People recovered by one plentiful Bleeding, and taking the mild cooling Medicines, fuch as the *mixtura e fpermate ceti cum nitro*, the faline or mindereri Draughts, or fuch like. When the Fever and Difficulty of Breathing continued after the firft Bleeding, in a Day or two a Vein was opened a fecond Time ; and immediately after a Blifter was applied to the Back, which commonly removed the Fever, and relieved the Breathing.—When the Patients were inclined to be coftive, a Dofe of Phyfic was of Service.

None of the *Britifh* died, except one or two of the Soldiers, who remained in Quarters after
being

being taken ill; and, inftead of bleeding and living low, indulged in the Ufe of fpirituous Liquors; and were not brought to the Hofpital, till they were in the laft Stage of a Peripneumony.—Many of the Inhabitants of the Town died of this Diforder, which was probably owing to Want of Care.

O F

OF THE

RHEUMATISM.

THE Rheumatifm is one of the Diforders moſt generally to be met with in military Hoſpitals. There were at all Times ſome Men in our Hoſpitals labouring under Rheumatic Fevers, or other rheumatic Complaints; though we never had at any one Time a great Number; owing probably to the Weather being very favourable in both the Campaigns of 1761 and 1762.—It was always moſt frequent when the Weather was wet and cold; both during the Campaign, and when we were in Winter Quarters.

It

It commonly began either, 1. With an
acute Fever, and Pains all over ther Body: or,
2. With Pains in particular Parts, as the
Shoulders, Legs, Arms, Knees, and sometimes
of the Side, attended with some Degree of a
Fever.—The first was the most common Form
it assumed, when Men were attacked with it in
the Field or in Garrison; owing to their doing
Duty in cold wet Weather.—The other Causes
generally took place when they had been formerly subject to rheumatic Complaints, and
had caught Cold; or after they had been weakened and reduced low by Fevers, Fluxes, or
other Diforders.

We had but very few Rheumatisms accompanied with Swelling, Pain, and Inflammation
of the Joints of the Knees and Wrists, &c.
which are fo common in our Hofpitals about
London. I did not meet with above a Dozen
Cafes, of this Kind, whilst in *Germany* with the
Army.

When the Rheumatifm began with Pains all
over the Body, attended with a High Fever, we
treated it at first entirely as an Inflammatory
Fever,

Fever (*a*). We blooded freely, and repeated
this Evacuation often (*b*), if the Blood continued fizy, and the Pains violent; provided the
Pulfe was ftrong. When the Pleura, the
Lungs, or any other of the Vifcera were affected, we blooded as freely as we fhould have
done in acute Inflammations of thefe Parts:

(*a*) *Sydenham,* in treating of this Difcafe, orders Bleeding,
and that to be repeated next Day; and afterwards every other
Day, two, three, or foar Times, or more, as the Patients
Strength can bear it; and on the intermediate Days to give a
purgative Clyfter. But in young People, and thofe who have
lived regularly, he fays, that a very low Diet will cure as effectually as Bleeding and Medicines: That the Patients muft
live four Days on Whey alone, but after this may eat Bread for
Dinner; and on the laft Days for Supper alfo; and when the
Symptoms begin to abate, he allows them to eat boiled Chicken,
or other light Food; but fays they muft live every third Day
on Whey, till their Strength returns. *Procefſ. Integr. de Rheu-
matifmo.*

(*b*) A Remark of Dr. *Huxham*'s deferves to be taken Notice
of here: He tells us, that there are fome Kinds of Rheumatifms,
viz. thofe which come from a fharp ferous Rheum, which do
not bear the free Ufe of the Lancet; that plentiful Bleeding
does more Hurt than Good; and that, in fuch Cafes, the Medicines which bring out breathing Sweats, and at the fame
Time correct the Acrimony of the Blood, joined with gentle
Opiates, have a much better Effect. *De Aere,* Vol. II. p. 185.

We

We gave the faline Draughts with Nitre (*c*) ;
and Plenty of Barley Water and other weak
diluting Liquors; and gentle Phyfic once or
twice a Week ; and afterwards applied Blifters,
which often relieved both the Pains and
Fever.

After fome Days, if the Pains ftill remained,
we continued the faline Draughts with Nitre
throughout the Day ; and in the Evening en-

(*c*) Dr. *Brocklefby*, in his *Obfervations on military Difeafes,*
recommends the Ufe of large Quantities of Nitre diffolved in
Water Gruel, or Sage Tea, (in the Proportion of two Drachms
of the Nitre to a Quart of the Liquor) in acute Rheumatifms.
He fays, " I am affured from numberlefs Inftances, that in
" ftout young Men, by taking fix hundred Grains (ten Drachms)
" daily, for four or five Days fucceffively, and diluting plen-
" tifully, as before recommended, plain Nitre proves the moft
" powerful and beft Sudorific, in fuch Complaints, that I have
" ever tried ; and this Quantity, and even more, may be re-
" tained in the Stomach, and pafs through the Courfe of the
" Circulation, by only diluting properly with thofe thin atte-
" nuating Beverages as before recommended. Such Quanti-
" ties, in three or four Days, feldom failed wonderfully to re-
" lieve the Patient, and very often to cure him entirely, by the
" moft plentiful and profufe Sweats." *See from p.* 116, *to p.*
124.

I have never hitherto given Nitre in fuch large Quantities as
here recommended by Dr. *Brocklefby.*

deavoured

deavoured to promote a free Perfpiration by
Means of the mild Diaphoretics, fuch as the
mindereri Draughts with Mithridate, in Dofes
frequently repeated ; at the fame Time, the
Patient kept in Bed, and drank freely of mild
diluting Liquors. Sometimes we gave twenty,
thirty, or forty Drops of Spirits of Hartfhorn,
in repeated Draughts of warm Barley Water :
or a like Quantity of the Antimonial Wine,
ufed in the fame Manner : or from fixty to a
hundred Drops of the Antimonial Wine, mixed with one-fourth Part of the *tinêtura the-*
baica, in a large Draught of fome warm Liquor ; which I have obferved, in many Cafes,
to have a better Effeêt, than moft other Medicines ufed for this Purpofe ; as it aêts both as an
Opiate in eafing the Pain, and procuring Reft ;
at the fame Time that it promotes a free Perfpiration, or gentle Sweat, to carry off the Diftemper.

But it fhould be obferved, that; in the Beginning of Rheumatic Fevers, forced Sweats
generally did Hurt, and often increafed both
the Pain and Fever ; and that in general we

had greater Succefs, and made fpeedier Cures, when we did not attempt to promote Sweating, till after other Evacuations had been fufficiently made, and the Fever had begun to abate; and that in this Fever, when we did attempt to procure Sweats, the milder Diaphoretics, with Plenty of weak diluting Liquors, anfwered better than thofe of a more heating Nature; though after the Fever was gone, and the Pains ftill continued, fometimes the ftronger Sudorifics, fuch as G. Guaiac, and its volatile Tincture, *Dover*'s Powder, and the like, beft anfwered the Purpofe, and carried off the Diftemper, when the milder ones had little Effect.

I have often obferved, where Sweating made no Change in the Diftemper, that keeping up a free Perfpiration by Means of the Decoction of the Sarfaparilla with the Antimonial Wine, or fmall Dofes of the *pulvis antimonialis* (*gr.* v.), given twice or thrice a Day, removed Rheumatifms, which had refifted the Force of other Remedies.

Some-

Sometimes the cold Bath (*c*) removed Pains which had not yielded to internal Medicines; but it ought to be obferved, that when Patients went into the cold Bath while the Feverifhnefs ftill remained, and the Blood continued fizy, or before free Evacuations had been made, oftentimes, inftead of giving Relief, it made the Diforder worfe, and more obftinate (*d*).

When the Rheumatifm was confined to a particular Part, attended with Fever, we treated it as the acute Rheumatifm. Fomenting the Part with warm emollient Decoctions, and

(*c*) I have frequently ordered the warm Bath with Advantage in Rheumatic Cafes in *St. George*'s Hofpital; but we had no Convenience of this Kind with the flying Hofpital in *Germany*.

(*d*) This I have feen many Inftances of, particularly in the Cafe of *Ann Walker*, a Woman of twenty-three Years of Age, who was under my Care in *St. George*'s Hofpital, in *May*, 1759. Before fhe came to the Hofpital, fhe had been blooded, and had gone into the cold Bath four Times, which, fhe told me, had increafed her Pains to a violent Degree; in which State fhe had continued for fome Weeks before fhe came to the Hofpital; but by being blooded, and taking the cooling faline Medicines, with gentle Purges, and mild Diaphoretics, fhe got well in a Month's Time.

L 2   ru bing

rubbing it afterwards with the volatile, or faponaceous Liniments, often gave Eafe ; and the Application of Cupping-Glaffes and Blifters frequently removed the Diforder. In fome Cafes, where the firft Blifter did not relieve, the Application of a fecond, and afterwards keeping up a Difcharge from the Part by Means of the Epifpaftic Ointment, carried off the Pain.   In others, where the mild Diaphoretics were ineffectual, Sweating, with the G. Guaiac, or *Dover*'s Powder, and fuch other Medicines, after the Fever was gone, removed the Complaints (*e*).

(*e*) Warm Water, pumped upon the Part, often removes fuch rheumatic Pains as have refifted the Force of internal and other Remedies.   On the 29th of *Auguft*, 1759, *Mary Ward* was admitted into *St. George*'s Hofpital for rheumatic Pains of the Arms, Legs, and Knees, attended with Fever, which all yielded to Evacuations, and the Ufe of cooling Medicines, mild Diaphoretics, and of the warm Bath, except the Pain of the Knee ; which, after it had refifted the Courfe above-mentioned, was at laft removed by pumping warm Water on the Part, three Times a Week ; joined to the Ufe of Fomentations and volatile Liniments.

When

When the Rheumatifm was attended with
Inflammation and Swelling of the Joints, we
blooded freely, gave cooling Purges, and the
faline Draughts with Nitre, along with Plenty
of weak diluting Liquors, and prefcribed a cool
low Diet.

After the Violence of the Fever and Inflammation was abated, fomenting the Parts, and
rubbing them with the faponaceous or volatile
Liniments, fometimes baftened the Difcuffion
of the Swelling ; as did likewife the Application of Blifters (*f*), after the Inflammation was
entirely

(*f*) *Ann Ragen*, a Woman about thirty-three Years of Age,
was admitted into *St. George's* Hofpital the 17th of *January*,
1759, for rheumatic Pains of her Legs and Arms, and a Swelling of her right Knee.   Free Evacuations, and the Ufe of cooling Medicines, and mild Diaphoretics, removed all her other
Complaints, except the Swelling of the Knee, by the Middle of
February, when I ordered a Blifter to be applied to it; after
which the Swelling gradually decreafed, and fhe was difcharged, cured, the 20th of *March.*—*Rachael Hyde*, a Woman
twenty-four Years of Age, was admitted into *St. George's* Hofpital the 9th of *May*, 1759, for fimilar Complaints, which were
removed by the fame Means, all except the Swelling of the
Knee.   A Blifter was applied, and moft of the Swelling went
away, but returned foon after: It was at laft removed by the

Ufe

entirely gone ; but it ought to be noticed, that
if volatile Liniments or Blifters are ufed too
foon, they will fometimes occafion violent Inflammation and Pain (*g*).

Rheumatic Cafes of this Kind are often very
obftinate, and require a confiderable Length of
Time before they are got the better of ; and
frequently more or lefs of the ˉSwelling, efpecially of the Wrifts and Joints of the Fingers,
remains ever after ; and Patients, who have
once had the Rheumatifm in this violent Degree, are always fubject to Relapfes ; as are even
thofe who have had the Rheumatifm but
flightly.

Mercury (*b*) has been recommended in the

Ufe of the warm Pump three Times a Week, and drinking a
Pint of the Guaiac Decoction daily.

(*g*) I have fometimes oidered Leetches to be applied to fuch
Swellings (as recommended by Dr. *Pringle*), and found them to
be of Service ; and, at other Times, I have applied emollient
Fomentations and Poultices, which have given great Eafe to the
Patient. —1 have feen Setonsˉor Iffues, made near the Part af-
fected, afford confiderable Relief.

(*b*) Dr. *Mufgrave*, in his Treatife *de Arthritide Symptomat.*
p. 30, cap. ii. fect. 10, fays, he has known a Salivation, raifed
by Mercury, cure the Rheumatifm.

Cure

Cure of Rheumatifms ; but I never found it do
any Service by itfelf, except in Cafes complicated with venereal Symptoms ; though I have
often given it, and even fometimes gone fo far
as to raife a Salivation, where the Pains were
moft fevere in the Night ; and the Patient, at
the fame Time, thought he had fome Reafon
to fufpect a venereal Taint, though no external
Symptom. appeared. However, many good
Practitioners have recommended fmall Dofes
of Calomel to be given at Nights, and next
Morning a Purge ; in which Way, I think,
I have obferved good Effects from its
Ufe.

The Bark was frequently of Ufe in reftor-
ing the Strength, and removing thofe rheumatic Pains which remained after Fevers,.
and other Diforders ; but, in other Cafes, it
had little Effect.

When the Rheumatifm continues long, and
has taken deep Root, *Sydenham* (*i*) advifes to
bleed from Time to Time, at fome Weeks
Diftance ; which, he fays, will either entirely

(*i*) Vide *Sydenham. Opera.* fect. vi. cap. 5.

L 4   remove

remove the Difeafe, or bring it to that Condition, that the Remains of it will be eafily extirpated by an Iffue; and giving fome of the volatile Salts in *Canary* Wine, Morning and Evening. I have always obferved in rheumatic Cafes, which continued long, that, after free Evacuations, the Patients received more Benefit from a mild low Diet, continued for fome Time, and the Ufe of diluting Decoctions with mild Diaphoretics, while they took gentle Purges once or twice a Week, than from any other Remedies.

I have given Half an Ounce of Soap a Day, for a confiderable Time, in fome old rheumatic Cafes, in the Manner recommended by the late Dr. *John Clerk* of *Edinburgh,* as mentioned by Dr. *Pringle* ; and, I think, with Advantage ; but have not had fufficient Trials to afcertain the Merits of this Medicine.

Dr. *Sydenham,* in treating of the Rheumatifm, which he calls fcorbutic, fays ; that after it had refifted Bleeding, Purging, low Diet, and other Remedies, he has cured it by giving thrice a Day two Drachms of an Electuary made

made of *conferv. cochlear. horten. recent. unc.* ij. *lujul. unc.* i. *pulv. ar. comp. drachm* vi. *cum fy-rup. aurant.* q. s. drinking after it three Ounces of a Water drawn from *Brunfwick* Beer, and fome of the antifcorbutic Plants.

There is no Diforder which Soldiers are fo apt to counterfeit as the Rheumatifm, when ever the Duty in the Field is fevere; but while there is no Fever or Size in the Blood, or other evident Marks of the Diftemper, and the Men look healthy, there is always Reafon to fufpect Impofture.

O F

OF THE

Autumnal Remitting Fever.

THE Remitting Autumnal Fever, called by the Antients συνεχης, was alſo one of the moſt frequent Diſorders during the Campaign.

This Fever is obſerved in moſt Countries, after the Juices have been highly exalted by the Heat of Summer ; and People are expoſed to the Heats of Mid-Day, and to the cold Damps of the Night. We obſerve it every Year in the Neighbourhood of *London*, eſpecially among the labouring People, who work in the Fields, towards the End of Summer, and in Autumn ; but it is generally in a milder Degree than in Armies, where Men are more expoſed to the Viciſſitudes of the Weather.

As

As we go further towards the South, this, as well as other bilious Diforders, becomes more frequent.

This Fever is reckoned the endemic Diſtem-per of the *Weſt Indies,* of the Coaſt of *Guinea,* and other Places in the Torrid Zone; but in thoſe warm Countries it appears in a more vio-lent Degree; makes a much more rapid Pro-greſs; and proves far more fatal than in our cooler and more temperate Climate. And it is obſerved to be always moſt frequent and moſt fatal where a Country is covered with Wood, or is marſhy; and where there are fre-quent Fogs, and much ſtagnating Water, which corrupts by the Heat of Summer.

In *January, February,* and *March* 1761, we had none of thoſe Remitting Fevers at *Pa-derborn.* In *April,* ſome few of the Soldiers, on their Return from the Winter-Expedition into *Heſſe-Caſſel,* had Fevers attended with bi-lious Symptoms; but they were rather of the continued, inflammatory Kind, and tending to malignant, than ſuch as could be called re-mitting.

The

The firft Time that I faw much of this Feꞏ
ver, was among the Sick fent to *Bilifield* in the
End of *June* 1761 ; foon after the Army took
the Field. The Remiffions were fhort, and it
partook much of the Nature of the common
Inflammatory Fever ; and moft of them were
cured by the antiphlogiftic Method. A Day
or two before we left this Place, it began to
change into the Malignant Hofpital Fever,
from the Sick being too much crowded.

In the Middle of *July*, about Twelve Hundred Sick were fent to the Hofpital at *Munfter* ;
and about one-third Part were ill of this Remitting Fever. It did not partake near fo
much of the inflammatory Nature as at *Bili-*
field; the Remiffions became much more evident; and it was attended much oftener in the
Beginning with bilious Vomiting and Purging ;
and in fonie few the Diforder turned to a Dyfentery. About eight or nine had it changed
into the Hofpital Fever, from the Wards in
one of the Hofpitals being too much crowded ;
and in fome few the Diforder terminated in regular Agues. In *November* feverals were taken

ken ill of it in the Garrifon of *Bremen*, which moftly ended in a regular Intermittent, the endemic Diftemper of the Place. Towards the End of *December* we had none of thefe Remitting Fevers, the Diforders turning more to the inflammatory Kind.

In *June* 1762, this Fever began to appear again among the Sick, fent from the Army, to the Hofpital at *Natzungen*; and it continued to be frequent through the Summer and Autumn; and the greateft Part of thefe Fevers this Year terminated in regular Agues, moftly in Tertians, and were cured by the Bark; whereas the Year before very few terminated this Way.

This Diforder in the Beginning had commonly the Appearance of a continued Fever; and many had a Sicknefs and Vomiting, and threw up a Quantity of yellow Bile, mixed with the Contents of the Stomach. In a few Days, efpecially after Bleeding, the Remiffions became clear; tho' on its firft Appearance in *June* 1761 they were fhort, and rather obfcure; and it feemed ftill to partake a good deal of the

Nature

Nature of the common Inflammatory Fever, the Blood being very fizy; but as the Seafon advanced, the Remiffions became more evident, and the Paroxyfms more like thofe of an Ague ; and the Blood lefs fizy, tho' at all Seafons of the Year it had fome Appearance of an inflammatory Buff in this Diforder. The Sick were reftlefs and uneafy at Night ; but commonly felt themfelves cooler and lighter' in the Day-Time : and although they had no cold Fit, as the Fever came on at Nights, and many of them no Breathing Sweat, as they became cooler and freer from the Fever in the Morning ; yet the Fits were fo remarkable, that many of the Patients ufed to fay they had a regular Fit of an Ague every Night, or towards the Morning ; and fome few, that they had the Fit every fecond Night. As the Seafon advanced, the Remiffions appeared more diftinct. However, there was always a good Number in whom the Fever went on in a continued Form, through its whole Courfe, without any Signs of Remiffion ; tho' they had all the other Symptoms of this Fever. In a few

Inftances

Inſtances the Fever, after it came to remit, changed again into a continued Form.

The Heat in the Time of the Paroxyſms roſe high, and ſeveral were delirious during its Continuance (*a*) ; but were quite ſenſible in the Intervals, though never wholly without the Fever.

At the End of *July* 1761, four or five were attacked with a Bleeding at the Noſe, in the Time of the Paroxyſms, and became cooler afterwards ; but it did not prove a Criſis in any of them.

The Urine in the Beginning was commonly of a high Colour, though ſometimes it was pale and limpid : At firſt it depoſited no Sediment ; but when the Fever came to remit, there was often a ſmall Sediment after each Paroxyſm ; and as the Fever was going off, it let fall a Sediment in all (*b*).

Some

(*a*) I did not ſee the Delirium riſe ſo high, nor the Paroxyſms ſo ſevere, as in the Marſh Fever deſcribed by Dr. *Pringle.*

(*b*) Dr. *Hillary* ſays the Symptoms of this Fever in *Barbadces* were much the ſame as thoſe of the σιιηχης, or continued Remitting

Some at firſt were inclined to be coſtive; others had a Sickneſs and Purging; and feveral of thoſe who were coſtive in the Beginning, were in the Courſe of the Diſorder attacked with a Purging; and others, after ſome previous Complaint of the Stomach, were ſeized with both Vomiting and Purging. In general, after the Sick continued ſome Days in the Hoſpital, they were inclined to be looſe; which was a favourable Circumſtance, when this Evacuation was not ſo great as to be in Danger of finking the Patient. Some were attacked with a Dyſentery.

In this, as well as in moſt other Fevers, the Sick frequently paſſed by Stool Worms of the round Kind; and ſometimes they vomited them up, or the Worms came up into their Mouth or Noſtrils while they lay aſleep in Bed; and ſome towards the Height were afflicted

ting Fever in England; except only that the Urine in this hot Climate never depoſits any lateritious Sediment, nor very rarely in any intermitting or any other Fever, except when a Criſis happens that Way. *Obſervations on the Diſeaſes of Barbadoes*, p. 23.

with

with Deafnefs, which was commonly a favourable Symptom.

Moft of thofe ill of this Diforder had a yellowifh Colour of the Countenance, which went
off with the Fever. It was more obfervable in
fome than in others; in general, it was flight;
fome few became yellow all over (c); particularly one Man, in the Hofpital at *Munfler*,
who, after being feized with violent Vomiting
and Purging, Convulfions, and Twitchings of
the Tendons, and Hiccup, became yellow,
as in the deepeft Jaundice. This Symptom of Yellownefs arifes from a Redundancy
and Abforption of Bile ; and is fometimes obferved in other Fevers as well as this (*d*) ; for
while

(*c*) Dr. *Pringle* takes Notice of this yellow Colour or Jaundice. He fays, "fome grow yellow, as in the Jaundice. This was
" found more frequent during the firft Campaign than after-
" wards ; it was an unfavourable, but not a mortal Symptom."
Obferv. part iii. ch. 4.—*Hippocrates* mentions the Jaundice oc-
curring in Fevers, *Aphor*. iv. § 62 & 64 ; and he reckons it
a favourable Symptom in ardent Fevers, where it happens on
the feventh Day. See *Book on Crifes*'s, fect. 3.

(*d*) Does this Fever, when accompanied with this univerfal
Yellownefs of the Skin, approach to the Nature of the yellow

M   Fever while we were at *Paderborn* in *February* 1761, two Men were brought to the Hofpital in Fevers, attended with this Symptom. They were both delirious, with parched dry Tongues, flight

Fever of the *Weft Indies?* As I had fo few Cafes of this Kind under my Care, I cannot determine any thing about it from my own Experience ; but, from the-Accounts of others, I fhould believe them to be very different Diforders.—In the yellow Fever of the *Weft Indies*, the Blood appears quite loofe and diffolved, without the leaft Appearance of Size, even on the firft Day ; and the general Yellownefs appears on the third or fourth, with Signs of a total Diffolution, and gangrenous Diathefis of the Blood : Whereas, in the Remitting Fever of *Jamaica*, Mr. *Nafmith* tells us, (See Dr. *Lind*'s firft Paper on Fevers), there is always an inflammatory Diathefis of the Blood. The Yellownefs in both depends on a Redundancy and Abforption of Bile; but in the yellow Fever of the *Weft Indies*, the Bile is in a much more putrefcent State, and a great Part of the Cure depends on the early and fpeedy Evacuation of it.— In the yellow Fevers which appeared in *Haflar* Hofpital, which are taken Notice of by Dr. *Lind*, in his *Two Papers on Fevers*, the Blood was in quite a different State from what it is in the Yellow Fever of the *Weft Indies* ; the Blood drawn from two of thefe Patients became covered with a thick yellow Gluten, and the Serum was of the Confiftence of a thin Syrup, and of a deep yellow Tinge, and tafted bitter ; and in another who was bled two Days before his Death, it threw up the fame thick yellow Gluten, tho' the red Part below was quite loofe.

Twitchings

Twitchings of the Tendons, and other bad
Symptoms; and one of them had a continual
Vomiting and Purging. They both died, and
the Body of him who had the Purging was
opened. All the Bowels, efpecially the Colon, were tinged with a yellow Bile, and had
a flight Degree of Inflammation all over their
Surface ; the Gall-Bladder was diftended with
a very dark-coloured Bile; but no Concretions
were found in its Cavity, or in the bilious
Ducts; nor Mucus, or any other Thing obftructing thefe Paffages. The Surface of the
Lungs feemed flightly inflamed; and there
was a fmall Quantity of greenifh Serum in the
Cavities of the Thorax. I could not learn the
Hiftories of thefe two Mens Diforders, before
they were brought to the Hofpital; but, from
the Symptoms, was inclined to believe, that the
Fevers had been of the malignant or petechial
Kind; and that the yellow Colour was only
an accidental Symptom of it; for on one of
the Men we could perceive obfcure Traces of
dun petechial Spots on his Breaft and Arms;
and the malignant Fever was frequent at this

M 2 Time

Time among the Troops, and the bilious autumnal Fevers had ceafed long before.

I could not obferve any certain critical Days, or Periods, when this Diforder terminated.— Some, who had it flightly, got well in a few Days ; with others, it continued longer : Some continued long feverifh, and would feem cooler and freer from Fever for a Day or two, and then grow worfe again ; and many had repeated Relapfes.

Neither could I obferve any regular Crifis in this Fever. Sweat was the Difcharge which ofteneft proved critical. Many feemed to be relieved by a Purging ; but as the greater Part had a Loofenefs after fome Days, which continued often through the Diforder, without producing any very fudden Change in the Symptoms, it feemed to be a favourable Circumftance ; though it feldom carried off the Fever fo fuddenly as to be manifeftly critical. The Urine broke, and dropt a Sediment, for the moft part, as the Fever took a favourable Turn.

When

When this Fever proved mortal, it commonly affumed a continued Form ; the Tongue became parched and dry, the Patient delirious, with Twitchings of the Tendons, Hiccup, and other fatal Prefages; while others were feized with a violent Diarrhœa, or Dyfentery, which funk them irrecoverably.

In the Beginning, it was abfolutely neceffary to bleed the Patients freely ; and frequently to repeat the Evacuation, where the Symptoms required it. The Blocd was of a florid Colour, and commonly threw up more or lefs of an inflammatory Buff.

In thefe Fevers, we were obliged to have particular Regard to the firft Paffages, efpecially in the Beginning of the Diforder ; for they were generally loaded with bilious Humours (*e*) ; which, if fuffered to remain in the Bowels,

(*e*) According to Dr. *Hillary*'s Account of the Yellow Fever in the *Weft Indies*, which is attended with bilious Vomiting, it bears bleeding once or twice, but not a third Time, before the third Day, but not at all after that Time ; and after Bleeding a great Part of the Cure depends on carrying off as much of the putrid Bile as expeditioufly and fafely as poffible,

which

Bowels, were either abforbed, and increafed the
Heat and Fever, or brought on a violent Diarrhœa; and therefore, after Bleeding, we gave
a Vomit

which he fays is to be done by making the Patients drink freely of warm Water (fometimes mixed with a little fimple Oxymel or Green Tea) fo as to vomit feven or eight Times; and
then to give a grain, or a Grain and a half of Opium, to procure Reft, and to fettle the Stomach; to make the Patient take
nothing for two Hours after; and then, if he has not had a
Stool, to give a laxative Clyfter; after fix Hours Reft, to
give a gentle Purge, to carry off as much as poffible of the
bilious corrupted Humours; and in the Courfe of the Diforder
to repeat the Purge, as often as the Patient is attacked with
an Anxiety, and a painful burning Heat about the Præcordia;
which almoft depend on bilious corrupted Humours pent up
within the Bowels; and to endeavour to fupport 'the Patient's
Strength, and ftop the putrefcent Diathefis of the Fluids by
fuitable Antifeptics, of which he found a watery Infufion of
Snake Root, mixed with *Madeira* Wine and Syrup of Poppies,
to anfwer the beft of any Thing he tried, and to fit eafieft on
the Stomach; and to this he added the Ufe of Cordials, and
of ftrong Wine Whey as the Patient became lower.

Dr. *Hillary*'s Purge was: R. Mannæ fefcunc vel unc. ij.
Tamarind. cond. unc. i. Tartar vitriolat. gr. x. folve in feri
laƈtis præparat. cum Vin. Maderienf. unc. vi. Colaturæ adde
Tinƈt. Senæ unciam dimidiam. Divide in Partes quatuor, &
capt. æger unam omni hora donec laxetur alvus.

His

a Vomit in the Evening, and next Day a Dofe of fome gentle Purge, as Rhubarb or Salts; to carry off thefe putrid, bilious Humours: And afterwards, in the Courfe of the Diforder, if the Patient was coftive, and grew hot, reft-lefs, and uneafy, we either repeated the Purge, or gave laxative Clyfters, which generally re-

His Infufion of Snake-Root was prepared in the following Manner:

R. Rad. Serpent. Virgin. drachm. ij. Croci Angl. drachmam dimidiam, infunde per horam vafe claufo in aq. bull. q. s. & dein unc. vi. Colaturæ, adde aq. Menth. fimp. unc. ij. Vin. Maderienfis, unc. iv. Syrup. Croci vel Syr. e Mecon. unc. i. Elix. Vitriol. acid. q. s. ad gratum faporem M. capiat æger cochlear. ij. vel iij. omni hora vel fecunda quaq; hora vel fæpius pro re nata.

The Stomach is fo irritable in the Beginning of this Difor-der, as to rejeft the faline Draughts, Nitre, and fuch other Me-dicines. Nor will the Bark, which might be judged a very proper Medicine in the fecond Stage of the Diforder, lie upon the Stomach, but is thrown up immediately, in whatever Form it is given. However, a Gentleman who had praftifed long in the *Weft Indies* told me, that although the Patient could not retain it in his Stomach, yet that he had found great Service, after the Bowels were emptied, from the Bark ufed freely in Clyfters.

Dr. *Hillary* difapproves of the Ufe of Blifters in the advanced State of thefe Fevers.

M 4   moved

moved thefe Symptoms.—Frequently after the
Operation of the Emetic, the Patient had fome
loofe Stools, from the Gall Bladder's being
emptied in the Strainings to vomit. Such Stools
were always bilious, as were commonly thofe
procured by purgative Medicines.

After emptying the Bowels, we gave the
cooling, and mild Daphoretics, fuch as the
faline and mindereri Draughts, joined occafionally with Nitre, or the Contrayerva
Powders; while we made the Patient drink
plentifully cf warm diluting Liquors ; which
we found to anfwer in general better than any
other Remedies: They brought the Remiffions to be mofe evident, and the Paroxyfms to
be milder, at the fame Time that they kept up
a free Perfpiration, as a Means to carry off the
Diftemper.

In fome Cafes we gave the Antimonial
Powder, made of one Part of Tartar Emetic,
and ten of the *pulvis e chelis*, in fmall Dofes,
from two to four Grains every four or fix Hours.
The firft Dofes of this Powder fometimes made
the Patient fick, and acted as a Purgative, and
kept

kept up a free Perfpiration ; at other Times, it produced no vifible Effect.   In fome Cafes, where it was given early, it operated both by Stool, and as a Diaphoretic, and removed the Fever (f) ; and it was of Ufe in others, towards the

(f) Dr. *Millar*, one of the Phyficians to the Army, told me in *Germany*, that he had given this antimonial Powder with great Succefs in the Remitting Fever, while the Eighth Regiment of Foot (to which he was formerly Surgeon) lay in *England*.—Dr. *Pringle*, in his fourth Edition of his *Obfervations*, Part iii. ch. iv. tells us, that having given a mild Purge immediately after Bleeding, he next Morning, when there was almoft always a Remiffion, gave a Grain of the Tartar Emetic, with twelve Grains of Crabs-Eyes, and repeated the Dofe in two Hours, if the firft had little or no Effect ; at any Rate, in four Hours.   This Medicine not only vomited, but generally opened the Body, and raifed a Sweat.   By thefe Evacuations, the Fever was fometimes quite removed, but always became eafier.—This Medicine he ufually repeated the fecond or third Day ; if not, he opened the Body with fome mild Laxative, or a Clyfter ; and continued this Medicine, till the Fever went gadually off, or intermitted.—Dr. *Pringle* fays, that Dr. *Huck* treated this Fever in a Method fimilar to this, both in *North America* and in the *Weft Indies*.   In the Beginning he let Blood ; and in the firft Remiffion, gave four or five Grains of Ipecacuana, with Half a Grain of Tartar Emetic : This Medicine he repeated in two Hours, taking Care that the Patient fhould not drink before the fecond Dofe ; for by that Means the Medicine paffed

the Decline of the Fever; but we were often obliged to lay it afide; for it either acted too roughly, or produced no vifible Effect or Alteration in the Diforder.

When the Fever came to remit, we were obliged, for the moft part, to continue the Ufe of the mild Diaphoretics, as before; for, although the Diforder put on a remitting Form, the Bark had very little Effect in ftopping it (*g*), unlefs

paffed more readily into the Bowels, before it operated by vomiting. If, after two Hours more, the Operation either Way was fmall, he gave a third Dofe; which commonly had a good Effect in carrying off the Bile; and then the Fever either went quite off, or intermitted fo far as to admit the Bark. On the Continent he found no Difficulty after the Intermiffion; but in the Iflands, unlefs he gave the Bark upon the firft Intermiffion, though imperfect, the Fever was apt to affume a continual and dangerous Form. Dr. *Huck* never varied this Method, but upon a ftronger Indication to purge, than to vomit. In which Cafe he made an eight Ounce Decoction, with Half an Ounce of *Tamarinds*, two Ounces of *Manna*, and two Grains of *Emetic Tartar*; and dividing this into four Parts, he gave one every Hour, till the Medicine operated by Stool.

(*g*) Dr. *Hillary*, in mentioning the Remitting Fever of the Ifland of *Barbadoes*, fays: In thofe who were blooded, and took an Emetic afterwards, and then the faline Draughts, the
Fever

unlefs where the Fever changed into a regular
Quotidian or Tertian Ague.——In the Year
1761, very few of thefe Fevers turned to regular Intermittents; but, in the Year 1762, the
greater Part of them terminated in regular
Agues, and were cured by the Bark (*b*).

In

Fever was generally carried quite off by a critical Sweat on the
feventh or ninth Day; in fome few it came to intermit regu-.
larly after that Time; and was foon cured by the *cortex Peruvi-*
ana, given with the faline Draughts, and feldom effe&ually
without them; though thefe irregular ingeminated Fevers often
remitted, and fometimes feemed to intermit; yet if the *cortex*
Peruviana was given too foon in the Difeafe, before it intermitted regularly (as I have more than once feen, where it had
been injudicioufly given), it generally caufed the Fever to become continual and malignant. *Obfervat. on the epidemic Dif-*
eafes of Barbadoes, p. 22.

(*b*) Mr. *Cleghorn*, after giving a very accurate Account of
Tertian Fevers, as they appeared in their various Forms of true,
of double, and tripple Tertians, and of Semi-Tertians, in the
Ifland of *Minorca*, tells us, that he firft attempted the Cure by
profufe Evacuations; but afterwards learnt from Experience,
that they were unneceffary; and that Bleeding and Purging
once or twice in the Beginning, was all that was in general requifite; and if on the fifth Day the third Revolution was not
attended with more threatening Symptoms than the fecond, and
the Patient bore it eafily, he frequently trufted the whole Bufinefs to Nature; which commonly terminated the Fever about
the

In the Year 1761, we tried the Bark in various Forms in many Cafes, where the Patient
had been blooded and purged in the Beginning,
and ufed the cooling Medicines; and where
the

the fourth or fifth Revolution; and for the moft part with an
Increafe of fome natural Evacuation.—But if the Paroxyfm on
the fifth Day was the longeft and moft fevere that happened,
attended with any doubtful or dangerous Symptom, he ordered
two Scruples of the Cortex to be given every two or three
Hours; fo that five or fix Drachms may be taken before next
Day at Noon; left, if this Interval efcaped, he fhould not have
found a favourable Opportunity of giving a fufficient Quantity
of the Medicine afterwards; as the Fits about this Period are
wont to become double, fubintrant, or continual.——This did
not always put an immediate Stop to the Fever, but it invigo-
rated the Powers of the Body, and prevented or removed the
dangerous Symptoms.   Having given the Bark on the fifth
Day, if a Fit came on the fixth, and declined the fame Evening, he gave fome more Dofes of the Bark to mitigate the Fit
on the feventh; yet fometimes this Fit of the fixth united with
that of the feventh, and the Patient had the Heat, Reftleffnefs,
Raving, and other Complaints, greatly augmented, and the
Cafe feemed more defperate than ever; which, however, were
more dangerous in Appearance than Reality, and went off with
a profufe Sweat next Morning; after which he gave the Bark
freely as before; and this either ftopt the Fits, or made them fo
moderate, as that they yielded quickly to the fame Sort of Management.—By this Method, when Affiftance is called timely,
Mr. *Cleghorn* fays, the moft formidable Intermitting and Remitting

the Remiſſions were very clear : Yet it had no
Effect in removing the Diſorder, except in two
or three Caſes at *Munſter*, where the Paroxyſms aſſumed a tertian Form ; for the moſt
part, it made the Patients more hot and feveriſh, and we were obliged to leave off uſing it,
as it was in Danger of changing the remittent
into a continued Fever. However, it was of
Service after the Fever came to a Criſis, and
was going off ; and Dr. *Pringle* has very juſtly
obſerved, that it haſtened the Recovery, and
that thoſe who uſed it were leſs ſubject to Relapſes than ſuch as did not ; and therefore we
commonly gave it in a convaleſcent State.—
Before giving the Bark, I always found it of
Advantage to give a Doſe of Rhubarb, or of
ſome other Purgative, or to mix ſome Rhubarb
with the firſt Doſes, ſo as to procure the Patient ſome looſe Stools.

When either the Fever went on without
Intermiſſion, or changed into a continued

ting Tertians, may be certainly and ſpeedily brought to a happy
Concluſion about the End of the firſt Week, or Beginning of
the ſecond. See *Obſerv. on the epidemic Diſeaſes in Minorca,*
chap. iii. p. 187, &c.

Form,

Form, or the Patient continued hot and feverifh through the Day, with a Head-Ach, and
other feverifh Symptoms, nothing anfwered
better, after free Evacuations had been made,
than to apply a large Blifter to the Back; and
to make the Patient drink freely of cooling diluting Liquors; which generally relieved the
Head, and abated the Violence of the other
Symptoms.

When a Purging came on in the Courfe of
this Diforder, if there was much Fever, with a
ftrong throbbing Pulfe, Gripes and Pain of
the Bowels, fome Blood was taken away; and
immediately after the Patient took a Dofe of
Salts and Manna, or of Rhubarb; and an Opiate in the Evening after its Operation : But if
there was little or no Fever, or fharp Pain,
Bleeding was omitted; and if the Patient complained of Sicknefs, a few Grains of Ipecacuana were given previous to the Purge.

After this, if the Purging was moderate, and
did not fink the Patient, we did nothing to
ftop it ; but if it was violent, we gave the mindereri Draughts with Mithridate, and the Chalk
Julep

Julep in the Day, and an Opiate at going to Reft; and occafionally ufed the emoilient and anodyne Clyfter; and, if neceffary, repeated the Emetic and Purge.

The Hiccup feldom appeared in this Fever till the Patient was reduced very low, and was commonly the Forerunner of Death. Some few, who had a Purging and Vomiting, were taken with a Hiccup, attended with Sicknefs, and Load at the Stomach, which feemed to depend on bilious Humours lodged in the Stomach and Bowels. This induced me to give a few Grains of the Ipecacuana; and to make the Patients drink an Infufion of Camomile Flowers till they vomited freely, and afterwards to take fome mild Purge, or ufe laxative Clyfters; after which they found themfelves eafier, and an anodyne Draught, with twenty or twenty-five Drops of the *tinctura thebaica*, put an End to the Hiccup. Others required the Ufe of Cordial Draughts, mixed with Opiates; and repeated Clyfters and Fomentations, before they found Relief. ——
The Application of a Blifter removed the Hic-
cup

cup in one, after the above Remedies had proved ineffectual; as did the Musk Julep with Opium, and the Application of an aromatic Plaifter to the Stomach, in another Patient.

Several of them complained of a burning Heat and Pain in making Water; which commonly went off by drinking freely of the Gum Arabic Decoction, with the dulcified Spirit of Nitre, and the Ufe of oily Draughts; though in fome it required the Affiftance of Opiates, and of Fomentations and Clyfters, before it was got the better of.

The Symptom of Worms we were often obliged to neglect till the Fever was over, and then we treated it as formerly mentioned.

The Deafnefs, though not near fo frequent in this as the Malignant Fever, was rather a favourable Symptom, and moftly went away of itfelf; though in a few Cafes, where it continued long, we applied Blifters behind the Ears, or to the Neck, with Advantage.

Many, efpecially thofe who were brought low, complained, after the Crifis of the Fever, of Reftleffnefs, and Want of Sleep; which, however,

however, went off as their Strength returned :
Where it fatigued them much, and kept them
low, we gave a Cordial anodyne Draught at
Night ; and if that did not anfwer, commonly
the Addition of a few Glaffes of Wine in the
Afternoon had the defired Effect.

Others, in their convalefcent State, complained of fuch a Giddinefs, and Lightnefs of the
Head, that they could neither walk nor ftand ;
others, of a Dimnefs of the Eyes. Thefe
Symptoms, for the moft part, went off as the
Patients gathered Strength : The Ufe of the
Bark, with now and then a Glafs of Wine,
haftened the Cure ; and in two or three Cafes
we were obliged to give a Dofe or two of fome
gentle Phyfic, and to apply a Blifter, before the
Patient got the better of them.

As the Sick were recovering, it was common
for them to complain of Pains of the Shoulders, Arms, and Legs, which alfo left them as
they recovered their Strength ; where they did
not, the faline Draughts, and a low Diet, generally had a good Effect ; and where it had not,
we treated them as rheumatic Complaints.

N   When

When the yellowifh Colour of the Countenance remained after the Fever, we kept the Patient on a low Diet; and his Body open by Means of the faline Draughts, with a few Grains of Rhubarb, or by giving Half a Drachm, or two Scruples of the Soap Pills with Rhubarb daily; which, for the moft. part, removed the Yellownefs foon. Two only had a Jaundice remain after the Fever, and both were cured in a fhort Time.

In other Refpects, the Treatment of this Fever, when it degenerated into a continued Form, had nothing particular in it; nor differed from the common Practice of giving cooling Medicines when the Fever was high, and fupporting Nature by the Ufe of Cordials and Wine, and the Application of Blifters, &c. when low; and promoting fuch Evacuations as Nature pointed out for a Crifis.

O F

OF THE

Intermitting Fever, or Ague.

THIS Diforder belongs to the fame Tribe
of Difeafes as the Remitting Fever. We
call it an Intermitting Fever, or Ague, when
the Paroxyfms are diftinct, begin with a cold
and hot Fit, and go off with a Sweat; and the
Patient is cool, and free from the Fever in the
Intervals between the Fits.

Many have been the Caufes alledged to produce this Diforder. The great Quantity of
Bile that is often thrown up in the Fit, has
caufed it to be ranked among the bilious Difeafes; and the Seafons of the Year in which
it is moft frequent, and the low moift Situation
of the Places where it is endemic, have made
Practitioners fufpect, that an obftructed Perfpi-

ration,

ration, and a Tendency in the Juices to the Putrefcent, are the Caufe of it.

But whatever Caufe we may fuppofe to give Rife to the firft feverifh Fit, it is difficult from hence to account for the regular Returns of the Paroxyfms and Intermiffions : For my own Part, after confidering Intermittents, which obferved a regular *Type* in the Courfe of a Salivation (*a*) ; their being fo eafily ftopt by the Bark without any fenfible Evacuation ; their being fometimes put away by a Stimulus exter- nally applied (*b*), or by a Fright, or fudden Plunge into cold Water (*c*) ; their ·returning

(*a*) See *Van Swieten*, Vol. II. p. 537.

(*b*) A Gentleman told me, that he was once cured of an Ague in the Country, by applying a Poultice of Garlic to his Wrifts, and letting it lie on till it inflamed and bliftered the Part.—I have feen Blifters cure an Ague.—In the *Edinburgh Med. Effays,* Vol. II. Art. v. we have an Account of Agues being cured by the Application of Poultices of recent Erigerum (Groundfel) applied to the Stomach on the Days free from the Paroxyfm, which caufed ftrong Vomiting.

. (*c*) See an Account of an Ague being cured by the Patient being pufhed into a Pool of Water without any previous No- tice, and being much frightened, in *Mafon's Account of Agues,* p. 222.

after

after flight Errors in Diet, and fometimes by the Operation of a Purge, or of Bleeding; .their attacking fometimes only particular Parts, and many fuch Accidents in thefe Fevers, I muft confefs, that I am unable to form any Idea, either of their Origin, Seat, or Caufe (*d*).

The Soldiers were fubject to this Diforder, particularly in Spring, if they took the Field foon, and in Autumn: The Frequency of it was in a great Meafure determined by the Nature of the Ground on which they were encamped, or the Situation of the Garrifon or Town in which they were quartered; for the lower and moifter the Camp or Garrifon, and the more

(*d*) The common Account given of the Caufe of Agues, and of the regular Return of their Paroxyfms, has been: That the Ague takes its Rife from fome Sort of Matter, bilious, or whatever it may be, either mixed with the Blood, or lodged in the Bowels, or in fome other Part of the Body; that a great Part of this Matter is thrown out of the Body, in the Time of the Paroxyfm; but that fo much remains as ferves by Way of a Ferment to affimilate other Particles to its own Nature; which, when collected in a certain Quantity, produce a new Fit; and, according to the Time that it takes to produce this Quantity, the Diforder affumes the Form of a Quotidian, Tertian, or Quartan Ague.

N 3   moift

moift the Seafon, the more fubject an Army is to Agues; and the drier the Situation of the Camp or Garrifon, and the finer and drier the Weather is, the freer they are from Diforders of this Kind.

In Winter 1761, we had but very few Agues in the Hofpitals; but on the Return of the Troops from the Expedition into *Heffe-Caffel*, and during the Spring, fome (though not many) were attacked with Quotidian and Tertian Agues, and but very few with Quartans.—In *July* and *Auguft* they were more frequent, and accompanied with more bilious Symptoms.   At *Bremen*, during the latter End of Autumn, and throughout the Winter and Spring 1762, we had Agues of all Sorts, and many inveterate Cafes; and all this Spring, and during the Summer and Autumn, the Ague was the epidemic Diforder all over *Weft-phalia*, as well as among the Troops.

In Spring 1761, what Aguès we had were moftly Tertian, fome Quotidian, and but two or three of the Quartan Kind.   They were, for the moft part, mild, and yielded to the Bark.
—Some

—Some of them began in the Form of a continued Fever; but after Bleeding, and the Ufe of the cooling Medicines for a few Days, they began to remit, and at laft ended in regular Quotidian or Tertian Agues: Others, at firft, appeared in Form of Remittent Fevers, attended with a ftrong throbbing Pulfe; but changed to regular Intermittents by purfuing the antiphlogiftic Method of Cure; and fome from the Beginning affumed the Type of Quotidian or Tertian Agues, but often attended with a good deal of Fever, for the firft two or three Days; and fome had a flight Delirium in the Time of the Paroxyfms, and the Pulfe was not quite fettled in the Intervals. In fuch Cafes, where the Patient was ftrong, nothing anfwered fo well as to take away fome Blood; and to give the faline Draughts with Nitre till the Fever was moderated, before we gave the Bark.

In general, there is a Prejudice againft bleeding in Agues, after they become regular; but I have always obferved, both in *England* and in *Germany*, that where Patients are ftrong and

plethoric,

plethoric, and the Fever in the Paroxyfms rifes
high, or the Pulfe remains quick in the Intervals, that taking away more or lefs Blood, and
giving the antiphlogiftic Medicines in the Beginning, eafed the Patient, moderated the Fever, and made it fafer to give the Bark foon;
and I never faw the leaft Inconvenience from
the Practice; but, on the contrary, have feen
feveral Intermittent Fevers change into continued ones from the Neglect of this Evacuation;
and have feen Cafes where the Bark, inftead of
ftopping the Ague, rather increafed the Fever,
till the Patient was blooded, and had purfued
the antiphlogiftic Method for fome Time; after which the Bark had its proper Effect, and
put an End to the Diforder.

As foon as thefe Agues became regular, and
the Patient was quite cool, and free from any
Fever in the Intervals, we gave the Bark;
which foon put a Stop to the Paroxyfms, without the leaft bad Confequences; but, before
giving the Bark, we always took Care to empty
the firft Paffages by the Ufe of Emetics and
Purgatives, where there was no Symptom to
forbid

forbid their Ufe : In Cafes where the Patient
was weak, and the Fits fo violent as to make
it neceffary to ftop the Ague, before we had
Time to adminifter Emetics or Purgatives, we
added fo much Rhubarb to the firft Dofes of
the Bark as procured the Patient fome loofe
Stools, as recommended by Dr. *Mead* (e); which
did

(e) Mr. *Cleghorn*, while at *Minorca*, after Evacuations, gave
the Bark at the End of the third Period, as we obferved before;
but where the Fever had been neglefted till about the third or
fourth Period, or badly treated in the Beginning, and the
Bowels were inflamed or overcharged with corrupted Gall, he
was obliged to endeavour to palliate the moft preffing Complaints, and to watch Evening, Night, and Morning for a Remiffion, and then immediately to fly to the Bark, as the only
Remedy that could avert the Danger. If the Patient was
ftrong, he gave Half an Ounce of the Bark, with fix Drachms
of the *fal catharticum amarum*, divided into four equal Parts,
of which the Patient took one every two Hours ; the Effeft of
which was, that the next Fit was mitigated, and an Intermiffion
commonly enfued, in which the Bark was repeated without the
Purgative, to finifh the Cure. —But where the Patient was excef-
fively feeble, and there was a manifeft Rifk of his dying in next
Fit, he gave Cordials with the Bark, inftead of the *fal catharticum* ; and endeavoured to throw in fix or feven Drachms in
the Space of ten or twelve Hours ; he having found by Experience, that if a fmaller Quantity is given, the Paroxyfms come
on

did not prevent its ſtopping the Ague, at the ſame Time that it anſwered the End propoſed of carrying off any putrid Humours that might be lodged in the Inteſtines.

In *England*, Vernal, Quotidian, and Tertian Agues, frequently go off after Bleeding, and taking ſome Emetics and Purges, and the ſaline Draughts, and cooling Medicines, for ſome Time, without the Uſe of the Bark; but in *Germany* very few yielded to this Treatment, and we were obliged to give the Bark (*f*) before we could put a Stop to them.

In

on earlier than uſual, and make all Attempts to preſerve Life unſucceſsful. See his *Account of the epidemic Diſeaſes of Minorca,* cap. iii. 2d edit. p. 192.

(*f*) Sometimes, when Patients are reduced low by Agues, the Stomach becomes ſo ſqueamiſh as to rejeċt the Bark in every Shape it can be given ; in ſuch Caſes, when the Ague cannot be ſtopped by other Means, it may be adminiſtered with great Advantage in Clyſters, of which the following is a very remarkable Inſtance.—*William Hadderell*, a Lad ſeventeen Years of Age, in the End of the Year 1761, was attacked with a ſevere Tertian Ague, in which a Mortification came on his left Foot, and one-half of it dropt off; notwithſtanding, his Ague continued to attack him every ſecond Day, and the Sore continued

In the End of *July*, and Beginning of *August*, the aguifh Cafes we had at *Munfter* continued to be of the Quotidian or Tertian Kind. The greateft Part of them began in the Form of continued Fevers, tending more to the bilious Kind than the preceding Months, and many of the Sick had bilious Vomitings in the cold Fits; and the Agues we had in Spring, and during the Campaign 1762, were of the fame Nature, and required the fame Treatment.

nued running on the 12th of *October* 1763, when he was admitted into *St. George*'s Hofpital. He was reduced extremely low; and the Sore of his Foot looked fo bad, that it was at firft imagined he muft lofe his Leg. He was ordered fome Vomits, and a Purge, and cooling Medicines, and afterwards to take the Bark freely; but his Stomach rejected it, in whatever Form it was given. Other Means were then tried to ftop his Ague, but with no Effect, till the 7th of *November*, that I ordered two Drachms of the Powder of the Bark to be given him twice a Day in an emollient Clyfter, with Half a Drachm of the *tinctura thebaica*, which ftopt his Ague in three Days; and he had had no Return of it on the 28th of *January* 1764, and had recruited his Health and Strength, and the Sore of his Foot was greatly leffened. Dr. *Harvey* (who teaches Midwifery in *London*) told me, that he has cured Children of Agues by Bark Clyfters, after the Bark Waiftcoats, and other Means ufed, had proved unfuccefsful.

Thofe

188 Of the Intermitting Fever, or Ague,

Thofe Cafes, which began in the Form of continued Fevers, were treated as fuch till they began to have regular Intermiffions; they then yielded to the Bark.

Some were attended with the Dyfentery; and the Purging and Gripes were moft fevere on the Days of the aguifh Paroxyfms. In fuch Cafes, we were frequently obliged at firft to neglect the Ague, and to treat the Diforder entirely as a Flux. Where there was much Fever, the Patient ftrong, and the Pains in the Bowels acute, we ordered Bleeding; and after it a gentle Emetic, and fome Dofes of the faline oily Purge, or of Rhubarb; and gentle Opiates in the Evening, and other Medicines proper in the Dyfentery, till its Violence was abated, before we gave the Bark: though in fome Cafes, where the aguifh Paroxyfms were very fevere, and helped to increafe the Purging, and the Patient was in Danger of finking, we gave the Bark, notwithftanding the Flux ftill continued; and the Method we followed was the fame as that I formerly mentioned, where it was complicated with the Malignant Fever; which

which was to give the Bark, mixed with Diaſ-
cord, and Opiates, or other Medicines proper
for the Dyſenrery, in the Intervals between
the Purges.

By this Treatment, very often both the Flux
and Ague went off. However, it ought to be
obſerved, that unleſs the aguiſh Paroxyſms
were ſevere, and in Danger of ſinking the Patient, or that the Diſorder had continued for
ſome Time, and the Paroxyſms were diſtinct,
we ſeldom gave the Bark till the Violence of
the Flux was abated : And where-ever much
Griping and Pain in the Bowels attended the
Flux and Ague, there Bleeding as well as Purgatives were neceſſary, before exhibiting the
Bark ; which ſeldom or ever agreed with
them, till there was an evident *Apurexia*, or
Abſence of Fever in the Intervals between the
Fits. Where theſe Cautions were neglected,
the Bark generally made the Patients worſe ;
and we were obliged to omit it, till the Violence of the Purging was over.

Some Agues were accompanied with the
Jaundice, though not in ſuch a high Degree as
in

in the confirmed State of that Diforder; and
commonly in the Beginning the Pulfe continued rather quick, in the Intervals between the
Paroxyfms; and the Patients complained of
fome Degree of Sicknefs for the firft two or
three Days.   With thofe the Bark always dif-
agreed, till the Feverifhnefs between the aguifh Paroxyfms was gone; and we found, that
the beft Method of treating them, was to
bleed in the Beginning, if there was much Fever; and then to give a Vomit and Purge, and
to repeat them, if neceffary; and where there
was no Purging, to give the faline Draughts,
and other cooling Medicines; and to add a few
Grains of Rhubarb, or to give fo much of the
pilulæ faponacæ cum rheo, daily, as procured
one or two loofe Stools.

  After the Ague had regular Intermiffions,
and the Patient was quite cool, and without
Fever in the Intervals, if the Diforder did
not yield to the above Treatment, which
it feldom did, we then gave the Bark freely;
even though the flight icteric Symptoms ftill
remained; and it put an End to the Ague, and

removed

removed the Jaundice at the fame Time, with-
out the leaft Inconvenience to the Patient. In
fuch Cafes, we generally ufed to add a few
Grains of Rhubarb to the firft Dofes of the
Bark; or gave the Bark made up into Pills with
Soap, and added occafionally a few Grains of
Rhubarb.

Several of thofe who had the icteric Symptoms along with the Ague, had bilious Vomitings in the Time of the cold Fit; they found
themfelves fick, with a bitter Tafte in their
Mouth, before the Approach of the aguifh Paroxyfm; and many of them, though they took
Emetics, which operated freely at this Time,
yet did not vomit up the Bile; but the Sicknefs and bitter Tafte continued till the cold
Fit came on, when they vomited Bile in large
Quantities. In fuch Cafes, after the Ufe of
Emetics and Purges, and the Ague was
brought to have regular Paroxyfms, with free
Intermiffions, the Bark, given as juft now
mentioned, removed the Ague and icteric
Symptoms, without the leaft bad Confequences.

Many

Many Practitioners of great Repute have been prejudiced againſt the Bark ; and tell us, that the free Uſe of this Medicine often lays the Foundation of Obſtructions in the abdominal Viſcera, eſpecially when it has been given where there was an icteritious Colour in the Eyes and Countenance ; and that, in ſuch Caſes, we ought not to give the Bark till theſe Icteric Symptoms are gone. At firſt, I was very cautious of giving it under ſuch Circum-ſtances ; till meeting with ſome Caſes where the Paroxyſms were ſevere, and became more frequent, while the Patient was ſo low, as to be in Danger of ſinking under the Diſorder, I gave the Bark freely, as the only Remedy ca-pable of preſerving Life ; which not only ſtopt the Ague, but carried off the icteritious Symp-toms (*g*), and reſtored the Patients to perfect Health.

After

(*g*) This agrees with what Mr. *Cleghorn* remarks of Tertian Fevers in his *Obſervations on the epedemic Diſeaſes of the Iſland of Minorca*, who ſays, " where there is an icteritious Colour of the " Eyes, we are likewiſe told, that the Cortex ſhould not be ad-" miniſtred ; though, in my Opinion, it is for the moſt part " dangerous

After this I gave it freely, in the Manner above mentioned, to fome Hundreds, with great Succefs; and I never faw any Mifchief follow from ufing it: Indeed fometimes, where it was given rather too foon, it did not fit eafy on the Stomach, and made the Patients hot and reftlefs; but, by laying it afide, thefe Effects immediately ceafed; and generally, after a little Time, the Paroxyfms became milder and more diftinct, when the Bark was again adminiftered, agreed with the Stomach, and put an End to the Diforder; and I am now convinced, from Experience, that the Cafes in which the Bark has done Mifchief, or given Rife to Obftructions of the abdomenal Vifcera, are but very rare; and that thefe Mifchiefs moftly arife from the Obftinacy of the Diforder, and not from the Ufe of this Drug; for I have oftener obferved thefe Obftructions where little or no Bark had been ufed, than where it was given freely (*h*). What probably has given

Rife

" dangerous to delay it, after the firft Appearance of that
" Symptom." Chap. iii. 2d edit. p. 205.

(*h*) Dr. *Pringle* takes Notice, that thefe Obftructions hap-

O   pened

Rife to the Belief of the Bark's doing fo much Mifchief, is, that in *Holland,* and other low fenny Countries, where Agues are endemic, they are oftentimes extremely obftinate, and yield hardly to any Remedies; and if they are ftopt by the Bark, they often return foon after, and by their long Continuance give Rife to Obftructions of the abdomenal *vifcera,* which have been attributed to the Ufe of this Specific.

In fome few Cafes a Purging accompanied thefe icteric Symptoms, which we treated much in the fame Manner as when the Ague was complicated with the Flux; we gave Emetics and Purgatives; and the mindereri Draughts with Mithridate, throughout the Day, and Opiates at Night, if the Purging was violent; if it continued, accompanied with regular aguifh Fits, the Bark, with Aftringents, generally removed both.

pened as often without as with the Bark ; and therefore feemed to depend on the long Continuance and Obftinacy of the Inter-mittent.   *Obferv.* part iii. chap. iv. fect. 2. p. 179. 3d Edit.

In the latter Part of the Year 1761, and
during Spring 1762, we had at *Bremen* many
Patients in Agues of all Sorts ; as Quotidians,
Tertians, Quartans, and irregular Agues of a
very obftinate Nature. The Town of *Bremen* is large and well built, fituated in a low
fandy Plain, with the *Wefer* dividing the old
from the new Town ; generally a confiderable Part of the Environs is covered with
Water in the Winter, and frequently the
Wefer breaks down fome of the Dikes, and
overflows all the Country round ; and every
Time the River overflows its Banks, the Cel-
lars of all the new Town, and of that Part
of the old Town next the River, are filled
with Water. All the Year round, on digging
two or three Feet deep into the Ground, you
come at Water.

Agues are endemic in this Place, and great
Numbers of the lower Clafs of People are
afflicted with them at all Times of the Year,
efpecially in Spring and Autumn.

Some of the Sick fent down from the Army
were bad of Agues ; but the greateft Number

O 2   we

we had in Hofpitals was compofed of fuch as
took it in Town ; either from doing Duty on
the Ramparts, or from lying in bad Quarters,
or getting drunk and expofing themfelves to
Wet and Cold ; and many Men of the invalid Companies who had come from *Embden*
brought with them old inveterate tertian and
quartan Agues.

Moft of the recent Cafes were eafily cured
by the Methods already mentioned ; though
they often continued longer, required a greater
Quantity of the Bark to ftop them, and a
longer Continuance of its Ufe to make a Cure,
than at other Places, which were more dry,
and higher fituated.

The moft obftinate of the recent Cafes were
the irregular Intermittents, which had regular Paroxyfms, but where the Pulfe was not
fettled in the Intervals; which we were obliged
to treat as Remitting Fevers till the Paroxyfms
became quite diftinct, and the Patient was
cool and free from any Fever in the Intervals ;
after which they commonly yielded to the
Bark.

But

But many of thofe Agues which had continued for fome Time, efpecially with thofe
Invalids who came from *Embden*, or who had
brought on frequent Relapfes by their own
Irregularities, were very obftinate. With many the Bark had no Effect; and its Ufe per-
fifted in feeming rather to exafperate the Paroxyfms, and to do Hurt. Nor had almoft
any Remedy we tried a better Effect. We
gave the following Medicines to divers Patients; the faline Draughts and cooling Medicines; Infufions of Camomile Flowers and
of other Bitters; Dr. *Morton*'s Powders of Camomile Flowers, Salt of Wormwood, and
diaphoretic Antimony; Dr. *Mead*'s Powders
of Camomile Flowers, Salt of Wormwood,
Myrrh, and Alum; Alum and Nutmeg;
large Dofes of *fal ammoniac*; large Quantities
of Spirits of Hartfhorn; the antimonial Drops
and Powders; to fome we gave Emetics, both
in the Intervals and immediately before the
Fits. In fome we tried to promote Sweats
before the Approach of the Fits, by making
them drink freely of warm Liquors while

O 3   they

they kept in Bed, and took diaphoretic Medicines; and to others we applied Blifters.—But all did not put a Stop to fome of thofe Agues.

With fome the Diforder continued till it broke down the Crafis of the Blood, and brought on a general Relaxation of the Fibres; and the Patients became cachectic, and fell into Dropfies, or were feized with Diarrhœas, of which they died. Some had Obftructions formed in the Liver or Spleen, or other *vifcera*, and fell into the Jaundice and Dropfies, which carried them off.—In the Bodies, of feveral whom we opened, we found Indurations of the Liver and Spleen—in two of them Suppurations of the Liver—and in one, who had had the Ague at *Embden*, and had long complained of one of thofe Swellings towards the left Side of the *abdomen*, called the *Ague Cake* (*i*), the Spleen was fo much enlarged as to weigh above four Pounds.

(*i*) I have feen the dead Bodies of four People opened, who had thofe Swellings of the left Side, commonly called the *Ague Cake*, which had come after Agues; and in all the Swelling was owing to an Enlargement of the Spleen.

Some,

Some, whofe Conftitutions were worn out by thefe obftinate Agues, fell into Confump-tions and other pulmonic Diforders in the Win-ter, of which they died. One Man died in the cold Fit (*k*).

Where-ever the Ague continued long, and the Bark had no Effect, we were obliged to lay it afide, and to try other Remedies adapted to the prefent Circumftances of the Patient.

The mild Methods fucceeded beft ; giving the faline Draughts and gentle cooling Medi-cines to fuch as were ftrong and plethoric, and had the aguifh Paroxyfms violent ; and the gentle Aromatics and Bitters, or Cha-lybeats, to thofe of a weakly Habit, or whofe Fibres had been much relaxed, and their Con-

(*k*) The cold Fit is the moft dangerous Time of the Paro-xyfm, and the greateft Part of thofe who die of Agues die at this Time; one or two Inftances of which I faw in the Mili-tary Hofpital at *Edinburgh* in the Year 1746.—*Van Swieten* fays he has feen the trembling and fhaking fo great in the Time of the cold Fit of Quartans, that the Teeth have dropt out of the Head. *Comment. in fect.* 749. *Aphorifm. Boerhaav.* vol. II. p. 511.

O 4 ftitutions

ftitutions greatly injured by this or any other preceding Diforder.

During thefe Courfes, we gave at Times gentle Emetics; and if the Patient complained of Gripes and Purging, which they frequently did, in the Courfe of this Diforder, we gave a Dofe of Rhubarb, or of fome other mild Purge; and after it other Medicines proper for this Complaint.

By thefe Methods frequently the aguifh Paroxyfms became gradually milder, and at laft vanifhed. At other Times, after they had continued for five or fix Weeks, we again gave the Bark, and found it to have the proper Effect. With others they continued thro' the Winter, and went off of themfelves in the Spring. With others they ftill continued; and as no Medicines nor Time feemed to have any Effect in that Country, we recommended their being fent over to *England* for Change of Air, as the only Means likely to remove the Diforder.

Two Agues which had refifted the Ufe of the Bark were cured by Powder of Camomile-Flowers,

Flowers, Salt of Wormwood, and diaphoretic
Antimony; and one by the Ufe of the aluminous Powders, with Myrrh.—One Invalid,
who had long been ill of an obftinate Tertian,
on catching Cold, was feized with an Inflammation of his Throat, for which he was blooded, and took a mild Purge; next Day there
appeared a Swelling of one of the parotid
Glands, which we endeavoured to bring to
Maturation, by the Application of emollient
Cataplafms; after fome Days it went entirely away, without coming to Suppuration;
but as there remained ftill a Confufion of the
Head, and a Quicknefs of the Pulfe, a large
Blifter was applied to the Back, which continued running for fome Days; after it dried
up he fell into a Fit refembling that of an Epilepfy, and next Day had another Fit of the
fame kind; from the Time the Swelling firft
appeared till the Time he had the firft Fit, he
had no Ague, but it returned the fecond Day
after the fecond epileptic Fit; another Blifter
was applied, and he had no Return of the epileptic Fits, though his Ague continued obftinate

nate till *March*, at which Time he was fent to *England* (*l*).—About the fame Time the aguifh Fits of two others were ftopt by the Application of Blifters, though they returned in both foon after.

Excepting in thefe few Cafes, I found no Medicines effectual in ftopping thofe Agues, which had refifted the Bark when properly given, though we tried a vaft Variety in different Cafes. The *cortex cafcarillæ*, or *eleutheriæ*, was given freely, both in Decoction and Subftance, in four Cafes, which had not yielded to the Bark, but without producing any good Effect; we had not an Opportunity

(*l*) On the 29th of *Auguft* 1759, a Man (*Murdoch Brinnen*) about thirty Years of Age, was admitted into *St. George*'s Hofpital for a very large Swelling of the parotid Glands and neighbouring Parts, which had come three Days before, after a Fit of the Tertian Ague, which did not return afterwards. The Swelling was difcuffed by the Application of emollient Cataplafms, which were intended to have brought it to Suppuration. He had no Return of the Ague, nor did any bad Confequence follow the Difcuffion of the Tumour, and the Cure was completed by a few Dofes of Phyfic, and a Decoction of the Bark, which reftored him to his Strength, and carried off the little Heat and Feverifhnefs which remained.

of

of trying this Bark in more Cafes of this kind, nor in Fluxes, the fmall Quantity of it which had come from *England* being all expended.

A Soldier of one of the Regiments of Guards, who was admitted into the Hofpital for œdematous Legs, and the Remains of a very bad Flux, which he had had ever fince the preceding Autumn ; after being cured of the Flux, and moft of the œdematous Swellings, was feized with an intermitting Complaint in *February*. He had no regular hot and cold Fits ; but every fecond Day, after a flight Shivering and Cold, he was feized with Gripes and a Purging. In one or two of the Fits his Pulfe was very quick, and the Pain of the Bowels very acute and fevere; which obliged us to blood him, and give him a Dofe of the faline oily Purge ; after which we treated the Diforder as a Flux complicated with the Ague, and gave the Bark mixed with Diafcord, and gentle Opiates at Nights, and at Times gentle Purgatives; the Ague and Diarrhœa ftopt very foon, and in a few Weeks he got free of all Complaints, though he ftill continued weak,

till

till he was fent to *England,* about the Beginning of *April.*

Many, efpecially thofe whofe Conftitution
had been fhaken by this or fome other Diforder, complained of flatulent Swellings of the
Stomach and Bowels, which affected them either while the Ague continued, or foon after it
was ftopped, and were very troublefome and
uneafy. For the moft part, thefe Swellings
were removed by the Ufe of cordial Medicines mixed with the Bark, or a Courfe of Bitters, and fome Dofes of Rhubarb given at proper Intervals. In fome Cafes, where they were
attended with Sicknefs, and the Stomach feemed to be loaded, a Vomit gave Relief. Very
often thefe Symptoms continued for Weeks
after the Ague had left them, and did not go
entirely off, till the Patient recovered his
Strength.

In *February, March,* and *April,* 1761, feverals of the Soldiers in the Hofpital at *Paderborn* complained of periodical Head-Achs,
which returned in moft, every Day; in others,
only every fecond; and afterwards Cafes of
this

this Kind occurred at different Times as long as the Army continued in *Germany*. Thefe Head-Achs generally began in the Forenoon, were very violent while they lafted, and confined the Patient to his Bed for fome Hours. During the Pain, the Pulfe was quick ; but in the Intervals the Patients were quite cool, and without Fever. Sometimes, tho' not always, the Urine depofited a little Sediment as the Head-Ach was going off. Commonly the Pain was all over the Head, but moft fevere in the Forehead ; though fometimes it was confined to one Side only.

Thefe Head-Achs we treated entirely as Agues of the fame Type. When the Patient was ftrong, fome Blood was taken away, and afterwards we prefcribed an Emetic and Purge, and then gave the Bark liberally, which generally put an End to the Complaint, without any bad Confequences attending.

O F

OF THE

J A U N D I C E.

THE Jaundice, or a yellow Colour of the Eyes and Skin, occafioned by an Abforption of Bile into the Blood, was another Diftemper which appeared towards the End of each Campaign.

This Diforder, for the moft part, takes its Rife (*a*) from Calculi lodged in the biliary Ducts (*b*); and fometimes from a vifcid Mucus

or

(*a*) Obftructions and Scirrhi of the Liver have been affigned as the Caufe of the Jaundice; but as we have fo many Cafes of this Kind related where no Jaundice appeared, it is now much doubted, whether fuch Obftructions, which do not affect the Ducts, are capable of producing this Diforder.

(*b*) We have numerous Cafes in *Bonetus*, and other phyfical Obfervations, where Calculi have been found in the Gall Bladder, or Pituita obftructing thofe Paffages (*c*) ; and it may be brought on by a Tumour, or any other Caufe (*d*), compreffing thefe Ducts, fo as to prevent the free Flow of the Bile into the Cavity of the Inteftines.

The yellow Colour, or Jaundice, obferved in the Ague, and fome other bilious Diforders, feems to arife fometimes from Spafms of the Ducts ; or from too great a Quantity of Bile fecreted and abforbed into the Blood, which feems evidently to be the Cafe where large

der, and Ducts of People who have died of the Jaundice ; and I have frequently found two, three, and fometimes twelve, fifteen, or twenty, fuch bilious Calculi in thefe Cavities.

(*c*) Vifcid Mucus or Pituita, or vifcid Bile, has been obferved frequently to obftruct the Ducts. Dr. *Coe* fays, fometimes icteric Patients difcharge very thick Bile, almoft as vifcid as Bird-Lime. See his *Treatife on biliary Concretions*, chap. ii. where he has collected a great Number of icteric Cafes, in which the Bile has been found quite vifcid after Death.

(*d*) See the Cafe of a Jaundice in *Bonetus*'s *Sepulchretum Anatomicum*, tom. II. p. 326, where the Sides of the common biliary Duct were compreffed by an Enlargement of the Glands about the *vena portarum* ; and we fometimes meet with a Jaundice in pregnant Women which goes off after Delivery, and feems to have been caufed by the Preffure of the Uterus and indurated Fœces in the Colon. *Van Swieten* fays, he has feen this very frequently, vol. III. fect 9:8, p. 95.

Quan-

Quantities of Bile are either vomited or difcharged by Stool; a Proof that the biliary
Ducts are clear, and free from Obftruction.

In the End of the Campaign of 1760, after
a continued Rain for many Weeks, the Jaundice had been very frequent, and in a Manner
epidemical, among the Troops, for fome Time
before they left the Field; and in paffing thro'
Munfter, about the End of *December*, I obferved
feveral ill of that Diftemper in Hofpitals, and
met with a few Cafes of this Kind in the Hofpitals at *Paderborn* in *January* 1761; but during the Spring and Summer, we had only one
or two now and then fent to the Hofpitals for
this Complaint; though towards the End of
the Campaign it became more frequent, and
feveral were fent down to *Bremen*; and fome
of the Garrifon were likewife affected with it.
During the Winter not above four or five were
fent to the Hofpitals I attended, and but a few
to the flying Hofpital, during the Campaign
1762. It frequently appeared in dropfical
Cafes, depending on obftructed Vifcera.

Thofe

Thofe in whom the Jaundice was the original Diforder, and not complicated with any
other, generally got well foon; but where it
appeared in dropfical Cafes, depending on obftructed Vifcera, it was commonly fatal.

In the Beginning of this Difeafe, Patients
ufually complained of Sicknefs, Heat, Thirft,
and other feverifh Symptoms; and fome had a
Vomiting, and Pain of the Stomach, for a Day
or two before the Jaundice appeared; the Urine
was always of a deep Colour from the firft;
and about the fecond or third Day the Skin,
and the Whites of the Eyes, began to be tinged with a yellow Colour, attended with the
common Symptoms of this Diforder.

Such was the Manner in which the Jaundice began in thofe who were taken ill in Garrifon; but thofe fent us from the Army could
feldom give any accurate Account of their own
Cafes.

In the Courfe of this Diforder, the Sick
were inclined to be coftive, though fome few
had a Diarrhœa; feveral, who had been reduced by Fevers, or other Complaints, before the

P   Jaundice

Jaundice appeared, were attacked with violent Hœmorrhages from the Nose ; and two had like to have died of them before the Bleeding was stopped. The Hœmorrhages did not prove critical, but seemed to depend on a dissolved State of the Blood.

On the Patient's being first taken ill, if he was plethoric or feverish, or complained of Pain, attended with Sickness and Vomiting, some Blood was taken away. Next Day we gave twenty-five or thirty Grains of Rhubarb in a saline Draught, and afterwards the common saline and other cooling Medicines, till the Fever was abated. If the Pain and Fever did not abate, a Vein was opened a second Time, and a few Drops of the *tinctura thebaica* were added to the saline Draughts, while emollient Clysters were frequently administered, and the Stomach and Belly fomented with Flannels dipped in warm emollient Decoctions.

When the Pain and Fever were gone, we then gave a gentle Vomit in the Evening, and next Day a Dose of Rhubarb ; and afterwards

fo

fo much of the *pilulæ fapcnaceæ cum rheo* daily
as kept the Body open ; or the faline Draughts
with five or fix Grains of Rhubarb in each, or
fuch a Quantity as anfwered the fame Purpofe
as the Pills; and from Time to Time repeated
the Emetic (*e*) and Purge.

Moft

(*e*) Vomits are reckoned amongft the moft efficacious Remedies in this Diforder, and I have often feen good Effects follow
their Ufe.—*Janet Crags*, a Woman thirty Years of Age, was,
on the 21ft of *December* 1758, admitted into *St. Gecrge*'s Hofpital for a Jaundice of fome Months Continuance. Her Eyes and
Skin were not of the common icteric Colour, but of a dark
livid yellow, for which Reafon both fhe and the Nurfes termed
her Diforder the Black Jaundice. She at firft complained of a
Difficulty of Breathing, and a Weight and Oppreffion about the
Region of the Liver, for which fhe was blooded, took fome
Dofes of Phyfick, and the Soap Pills with Rhubarb ; but thefe
produced no Change in her Complaints. On the 29th fhe had a
Cough, and complained much of Sicknefs and Difficulty of
Breathing, for which fhe was ordered a Vomit, and afterwards
to take the Squill Draught Morning and Evening, which occafioned a Purging and Gripes. On the 5th of *January* 1759,
the Loofenefs ftill continuing, I ordered her to leave off the
Ufe of the Squill Draughts, and to take only fome Rhubarb in
an oily Draught every Night at Bed-Time. On the 8th, tho'
the Purging had increafed, I did not chufe to check it, as I fufpected it would prove a Crifis to the Diforder, and therefore
only ordered her the Cordial Draughts and Wine to fupport

Moft of the icteric Cafes we had, which were not complicated with other Diforders, yielded to the above Treatment in about twelve or fourteen Days. Two or three remained obftinate for a longer Time. To one I ordered a Quart of the pectoral Decoction, made with Parfly Roots inftead of the Linfeed, to be drunk daily along with the Soap Pills ; and the Jaundice difappeared in about eight or ten Days. One who had the Difeafe more obftinate than the reft, and complained for fome Time of a Tenfion and Uneafinefs about the Liver, was

her Strength. The Loofenefs continued till the 15th, when moft of the icteric Symptoms were gone, and by the 30th they entirely difappeared. However, fhe continued low, and fub-ject to Flatulencies for fome Months afterwards, which were at laft removed by the continued Ufe of Cordials, gentle Bitters, a nourifhing Diet, and repeated Dofes of Rhubarb; and on the 2d of *May* fhe was difcharged in a firm State of Health.

Dr. *Coe* fays, " I have more Reafon to be fatisfied of the " Effect of Vomits in diflodging thefe Calculi, than of any " other, or indeed of all other Medicines." *Treatife on biliary Concretions*, chap. ii. p. 253. Befides vifcid Humours, which Vomits bring away from the biliary Paffages, how often are Gall Stones likewife found in the Stools after the Operation of a Vomit? *Ibid.* p. 256.

ordered

ordered to have the right Side fomented Morning and Evening, and to rub it for fome Time
after with the *linimentum faponaceum*, and to
drink the Decoction of Sarfaparilla after the
Soap Pills ; and by continuing this Courfe for
about three Weeks, the Diforder went off (*f*).
The

(*f*) Sometimes the warm Bath has a good Effect after other
Remedies have afforded no Relief. In the Year 1743, a young
Gentleman, a Student of Phyfic at *Edinburgh*, had a Jaundice
for which he had taken Variety of Medicines, and rode daily
on Horfeback for fome Weeks, without receiving any Benefit :
At laft, by my Father's Advice, he took a brisk Dofe of Phyfic, and before it began to operate had a large Quantity of
warm Whey thrown up by way of a Clyfter, and went immediately into the warm Bath. In the Bath he was taken with a
violent Inclination to go to Stool ; and after coming out, had
a great Number of bilious Stools that Day, and next Morning
was ftill inclined to be loofe ; and in a few Days all the icteric
Symptoms vanifhed. On the 20th of *July* 1763, a middle aged
Woman, *Elizabeth Hofier*, was admitted into *St. George's* Hofpital for a Jaundice, which came about a Fortnight before. She
had been blooded, and had taken fome Medicines, before I faw
her. I ordered her a Vomit and Purge, and to take too Scruples of the Soap Pills and Rhubarb daily ; and four Days afterwards the Vomit and Purge were repeated, but without making any Change in her Diforder. On the 29th fhe went into
the warm Bath, and took a Vomit immediately on coming out.

The Hæmorrhage from the Nose commonly
ſtopped ſoon. Where it was violent, we kept
the,

After the Vomit ſhe had ſome looſe Stools, and the iſteric
Symptoms went all off in a few Days. She continued well for
ſome Months; but I have been told, that ſhe has ſince relapſed.

When the Jaundice continues obſtinate, there is hardly any
Thing has often a better Effeſt than the continued Uſe of De-
coſtions of the Juices of ſucculent Plants, of Whey in the Spring,
Soap, and ſuch like Medicines. The Baron *Van Sweiten* tells us,
that he has cured many obſtinate Jaundices by making the Pa-
tients drink daily a Pint or two Pints of a Decoſtion of Graſs,
Dandelion, Fumaria, Succory, and ſuch like, prepared in
Whey ; to each Pint of which he added Half an Ounce of *ſal
polychreſt*, and an Ounce or two of Syrup of the five aperient
Roots ; and by ordering them to drink the Spa Water in Summer, and take freely of Soap, along with a Decoſtion of the
aperient Roots, in Winter. In theſe who were cured by theſe
Remedies, he ſays, Stones, or a kind of a grumous calculous
Matter, were always found in the Stools, as the Jaundice was
going off. He relates one very particular Caſe of a Lady of
ſixty Years of Age, who had had a black Jaundice for twelve
Years, and was cured by continuing the Uſe of theſe Medicines for eighteen Months.; during the laſt ſix Months of
which ſhe had a Looſeneſs, and conſtantly diſcharged by Stool
a fetid granulated Matter of the Colour of Clay ;—and another
ſingular Caſe of a Man who was cured by living moſtly upon
Graſs, and a Decoſtion of it, for two Years together. The
Man came at laſt to devour ſuch Quantities of it, and could
diſtin-

the Patient cool, and applied Cloths dipped in Vinegar and Water to the Nofe.——In two Cafes, one at *Munfter*, the other at *Bremen*, the Patients were hot and feverifh, and a Vein was opened, and eight or ten Ounces of Blood taken away; and in one Cafe nothing took Effect till we gave repeated Dofes of the *tinctura faturnina* in a common acid Julep.

distinguifh the good Sort from the bad fo well, that the Farmers often ufed to drive him out of their Fields. Vol. III. §. 950.

· *Gliffon* tells us, that Cattle are fubject to bilious Concretions in Winter, which are diffolved and evacuated in the Spring, when they begin to move much about, and to eat the new Grafs, which purges them. *Oper.* vol. II. *Anat. Hepat.* chap. vii. p. 104.

Dr. *Ruffel* greatly recommends the Ufe of Sea Water along with the faponaceous Medicines. See his *Treatife on the Ufe of Sea Water.*

P 4 O F

O F

TUMOURS of the BREAST.

IN *May* 1761, a great many of the Patients, who had been in Hofpitals the preceding Winter, had Tumours formed on the external Part of the Breaft, which they fhewed me at *Ofnabruck*. They began in the Form of indolent Tumours, and came flowly to Suppuration. For the moft part, the Suppuration was only partial, and the Tumour, on being opened, difcharged a very fmall Quantity of Matter. Some of them, though they felt foft, and feemed to contain Matter, yet, upon being opened, difcharged only a fmall Quantity of black Blood. None of them melted down entirely into Pus, or came fully to Suppuration, and healed kindly as Abfceffes which fucceed acute

acute Inflammations. But after a fmall Quantity of Matter was difcharged, for the moft part, there ftill remained a hard Tumour, which felt as if it was a Swelling of the Bone, or Cartilage below; and in fome the Surface of the Bone was found rough at the Bottom of the Abfcefs.

Thefe Tumours feldom rofe high, and were moft of them fituated at the lower Part of the Sternum, or a little to one Side of it, commonly on the left Side, above the *cartilago enfiformis*. Some Patients had only one, others two, and fome three fuch Tumours. The firft of them I faw was on the left Side, which, on being felt, gave exactly the fame Senfation as when the Cartilages of the Sternum are begun to be raifed by an Aneurifm of the Aorta ; only no Pulfation was to be perceived ; and moft of them had the fame Appearance.

The Patients, who had fuch Tumours, commonly complained of Pains of their Breaft. One or two, after thefe Tumours came to Suppuration, feemed to recover their Health, and to feel no Uneafinefs, tho' fome of the Swelling remained :

remained : But many of them were inclined to be hectic, and feemed likely to grow confumptive.

Being ordered up to the flying Hofpital in *June*, and the Sick going down to *Bremen*, I had no Opportunity of feeing the Event of thefe Tumours, or of examining the Bodies of thofe who died with them. One I accidentally met with the following Winter at *Bremen*, who died of a Confumption and Diarrhœa. He had a large Abfcefs, which penetrated into the Cavity of the Cheft, and difcharged a great Quantity of very fetid Matter, at the Part where one of thefe Tumours had been feated, and the Sternum and Ribs were carious all round the Abfcefs.

O F

O F

PARALYTIC COMPLAINTS.

SOME of the Soldiers, from lying out in
the Nights on the wet Ground, and from
doing Duty in cold rainy Weather, were feized
with a Pain and Numbnefs all over, and loft
the Ufe of their Limbs, which in fome was fucceeded with a Palfy of thefe Parts : But the
greateft Number of thofe afflicted with Paralytic Symptoms were feized with them either
in Fevers, or after feverifh and other Diforders.
The Number, who were attacked with Complaints of this Kind, were but few.

When Men were fuddenly taken with Pain
and Numbnefs all over, we found that the beft
Method of treating them was to put them to
Bed, and give them Plenty of mild warm diluting

luting Liquors for Drink; and if there was
much of a Fever, to open a Vein, to give the
cooling antiphlogiftic Medicines, and apply
Blifters; and if thefe Complaints ftill remained, to endeavour to promote a breathing Sweat,
by means of Diaphoretics and warm Drinks.
Several who were brought to the Hofpital,
foon after being feized in this Manner, got
well; but in fome few, one or other of the
Limbs would begin to wafte, and remain paralytic afterwards.

Thofe who had the true confirmed Palfy
feldom remained long enough with us to be
cured.   Two or three received Benefit from
Blifters applied to the Parts, 'and from Iffues;
drinking at the fame time the Decoction of
the Woods, or of Sarfaparilla, and taking the
volatile Tincture of Guaiac or Valerian (*a*),
and

(*a*) On *Wednefday* the 1ft of *February* 1764, *Margaret Ju-
lion*, a Woman between fifty and fixty Years of Age, was admitted into *St. George*'s Hofpital for an entire Lofs of Speech,
which feemed to depend on a paralytic Diforder of the Parts
about the Larynx.   The Account her Friends who came with
her to the Hofpital gave of her Cafe was, that fhe had been
for

and being fweated by the Ufe of *Dover's* Powder, or other Diaphoretics.

One Man of the 51ſt Regiment of Foot, after doing Duty in very cold wet Weather, in the Beginning of the Year 1762, was feized with a Palſy of one Side of his Face, which

for five Months troubled at Times with Pains of her Bowels, and a Purging; that on *Sunday* fe'night before coming to the Hofpital, ſhe had fuddenly loſt the Ufe of her Speech, and had not fpoke fince that Time, though ſhe feemed to hear and underſtand whatever was faid to her. I aſked her fome Queſtions, which ſhe anfwered diſtinctly by Signs. She had no paralytic Complaint of her Face, Arms, Legs, or any other Part of her Body, and fwallowed both Fluids and Solids with Eafe. She had no Fever, and feemed to complain of nothing but the Lofs of Speech.—A Bliſter was applied to her Neck, and ſhe was ordered the faline Draughts, with a Scruple of Powder of Valerian in each, to be taken three Times a-day, and a Dofe of facred Tincture, to be taken twice a-Week. She followed this Courfe for a Fortnight, when another Bliſter was applied to the Fore-part of the Neck, and the Powder of Valerian in the Draughts was changed for two Drachms of the *tinctura valeriana volatilis.* At the End of three Weeks ſhe could pronounce the two Words *Why*, *What*. She continued the fame Courfe till this Day, the 16th of *March*, and can now pronounce many Words and ſhort Sentences.

prevented

prevented him from fpeaking diftinctly, and was an Impediment to his eating. He mended much after being blooded, and having a large Blifter to his Neck, kept open for fome time by means of the epifpaftic Ointment.

O F

INCONTINENCY of URINE.

AN Incontinency of Urine was another Complaint frequent among the Soldiers; but it seemed to me to be counterfeited by many. All, who had it, said that they had received some Hurt (*a*) or Sprain of the Back,

or

(*a*) A Soldier in the Hospital at *Paderborn* used to discharge his Water involuntarily, and mixed with Pus, which came from some violent Blows he had received on the Back.

John Pearce, a young Man about eighteen Years of Age, was admitted into *St. George's* Hospital, the 10th of *April* 1759, for a Pain of his Side, and a Complaint of the Bladder. The Account which he gave of his own Case was, that, some Months before, he had received a violent Blow with a Cricket-Bat on the left Side, en the Region of the Kidney; and that ever since he had had a sharp Pain in that Part, and sometimes had a Stoppage of Urine, and at other Times it came away insensibly.

or a Kick from a Horfe, or that a Carriage
had run over them.

Thofe

infenfibly. His Pulfe was rather quick, but low, and he had
a feverifh Heat. He at firft took fome cooling Medicines;
but on the 20th, being low and faint, he had fome of the
fœtid Julep. On the 23d he was attacked with a fharp Pain
in the Belly and Side, had a Stoppage in making Water,
a quick and full Pulfe, and moft of the Symptoms of the
Stone. He was ordered to be blooded immediately, to take
the faline Draughts every four Hours; and as he was inclined to be coftive, to take as much lenitive Electuary as to
procure him a loofe Stool; and it was recommended that he
fhould be founded as foon as the Violence of the Fever was
over. On the 25th he continued much in the fame Way, and
had made fome Water, which was intolerably fœtid. Half a
Drachm of the dulcified Spirit of Nitre, and five Drops of the
tinctura thebaica, were added to each of his Draughts, as the
Pain and Difficulty of making Water had increafed. On the
26th his Pulfe rofe, and became very hard and quick; the Pain
in his Side, and the Dyfuria, became more violent; and about
Twelve o'Clock he had a convulfive Fit, refembling that of an
Epilepfy; after coming out of the Fit, as the Fever and Pain
had increafed, he was blooded; the Belly was fomented and
embrocated, and he took the oily Draughts four Times a-Day;
his Blood immediately threw up a very thick Buff. He remained pretty eafy the reft of the Day; but about the fame
Time next Day, he had another convulfive Fit, and died.

On opening his Body, we found about two or three Pints of
a dark-coloured fœtid Water in the Abdomen; on cutting
through,

Thofe who really had the Diforder feemed
to have received fuch an Injury of the Bladder,
or Kidneys as required a confiderable Space of
Time to get the better of; and by reafon of
the fhort Time we had them under our Care
at the flying Hofpital, they feldom received

through, and fqueezing the right Kidney there came out a
thin purulent Matter every where from its Subftance, though
it appeared found ; on raifing and cutting through the Perito-
neum, covering the left Kidney; there was a Difcharge of about
a Pint of black and very fœtid Water, which had every where
furrounded this Kidney; and there were fix mortified Spots
on its Surface, as large as the End of one's Finger, with a
Depreffion in each about a Quarter or Half an Inch deep ;
molt of the Subftance of this Kidney feemed difeafed, and it
was full of Suppurations. The Bladder was contracted and
thickened, and contained a rough Stone, which weighed three
Ounces. The reft of the *vifcera* were found. This Stone had
certainly been in the Bladder long before the young Fellow
received the Blow with the Cricket-Bat ; but the Injury done
the Kidney had probably aggravated the Symptoms.

I do not remember ever to have feen convulfive Fits, fuch as
this young Man had, in acute Difeafes, except in one Cafe of
a flow Fever, which came by taking Cold after a Salivation,
and which I attended, along with Dr. *Pringle*. The Gentleman had three Fits exactly of the fame kind as this young
Man, at twenty-four Hours Diftance from one another, and
he died of the third.

Q   much

much Benefit.   One or two thought they grew better on taking the Bark and Balfam of *Peru* ; at the fame Time they bathed Morning and Evening the lower Part of the Abdomen and Perinæum, with Flannels dipped in gentle aftringent Liquors, applied cold.   Blifters applied to the *os facrum* had no Effect.

O F

OF A

STOPPAGE of URINE.

WE formerly mentioned, that in acute Difeafes many complained of a Stoppage or Difficulty of making Water; and others had this Complaint from Strictures of the Urethra, or Diforders of the Bladder or Kidneys (a).

Where

(a) It is often very difficult to judge of the Caufe, or to be able to determine exactly the Seat of thefe Diforders before Death; as the following Cafes will fhew.

John Waden, a middle-aged Man, was admitted into *St. George's* Hofpital the 10th of *April* 1759, for a Swelling of the Abdomen, and a Difficulty of making Water, which he faid begun about two Months before, with a violent Pain in his Back and Belly, occafioned by his being employed in making of Cyder in a very cold Cellar. He had not had a Stool for fome Days; at firft he took a Dofe of Phyfic, and fome of

Q 2

the

Where it depended on Strictures of the U-
rethra, Bougies introduced into that Paffage,
and

the faline Draughts ; but in a Day or two complained that his
Belly had grown to a monftrous Size, and that he had not
made Water for above twenty-four Hours ; on examining, we
found the Bladder fo much diftended as to reach up to the Na-
vel ; and upon a Catheter's being introduced, above two
Quarts of Water were drawn off, and the Swelling immediately fubfided ; but in the Afternoon was as large as before,
the Bladder feeming to be in a paralytic State. During the
Months of *May* and *June*, his Water was drawn off twice a-
Day ; he had his Belly fomented with emollient, aftringent,
and other Decoctions, and embrocated with Liniments ; was
blooded once when feverifh, took Cordials, the Bark, Myrrh,
and a Variety of Medicines, without any Effect. On the 3d
of *July*, a flexible Catheter was introduced into the Bladder,
and left there, in order that the Urine might drain away as faft
as it was fecreted, and the Bladder be allowed to contract, and
recover its Tone. The Catheter gave him no Pain, and he
thought himfelf much eafier by the Bladder's never being too
much ftretched ; but on taking out the Catheter fome Days
after, he had the fame Stoppage of Water as before. On con-
fulting with Dr. *Batt* and the other Phyficians, it was agreed
to give two Grains of the Powder of Cantharides, with three
Grains of Camphor and ten of Sugar, rubbed well together in
a Mortar, twice a-Day ; and to continue the Ufe of the flexible Catheter. He found no Uneafinefs or Strangury from the
Ufe of the Cantharides, and thought he paffed his Water more
freely, when the Catheter was taken out ; but after fourteen
Days,

and worn for fome Time, were of great Service. The Patients were at the fame time ordered

Days, finding no Change for the better, and being free from
any Fever, he was ordered into the cold Bath ; the two firft
Days he found himfelf more lively and brifk ; but the third
Day was chilly and cold after coming out of it, and therefore
was defired to leave it off ; fome Days after he became hectic,
and I obferved Pus in his Water, which he faid he had paffed
with his Urine for above three Months ; after this he languifhed for near a Month, and died upon the 25th of *Auguft*.
—Upon examining his Body next Day, we found the thoracic
Vifcera in a found State, except that the Lungs adhered a litt'e
on the right Side. Both Kidneys were difeafed ; they were
inflamed, and feemed enlarged ; and on cutting them, had
Tubercles difperfed every where through their Subftance,
which had come to Suppuration, and contained a good deal of
Matter ; the lower Part of the left Kidney was mortified, and
contained two or three Ounces of a black foetid Liquor. The
Bladder of Urine was contracted, and its Coats greatly thickened, and the internal Coat much inflamed ; and there was a
Cyft full of Matter, about Half the Size of a Walnut, between
the mufcular and villous Coats, towards the lower Part of the
right Side of the Bladder ; and there were two large Cyfts,
containing a fmall Quantity of Matter, though capable of containing near two Ounces each ; one fituated between the *veficulæ feminales* and Rectum, the other between the *veficulæ* and
Bladder, which opened into the Urethra by one common Ori-
fice, capable of admitting a large Quill, at the Side of the *ca-
put galinaginis*. The reft of the Vifcera were in a found State.

Mary

dered to live on a cool Diet, and to drink the
decoctum Arabicum, or an Infusion of Lin-
seed,

Mary Hibbcrd, a Woman twenty-four Years of Age, was
admitted into *St. George's* Hospital, the 6th *June* 1759, for a
Complaint of her Bladder. The Account she gave of herself
was, that, about *Christmas* 1758, she had parted with some
Gravel ; and about fourteen Days before coming to the Hospital, she was seized with a violent Pain in her Back and Loins,
attended with a Sickness and Naufea; and very foon after
complained of a violent Pain in the lower Part of her Belly,
and with a perpetual Inclination to make Water, though she
felt a sharp Pain and Difficulty in doing it; and that these
Complaints still remained. Her Pulse was quick and strong,
and she was inclined to be costive. She was immediately
blooded, took the oily Draughts three Times a-Day, the *decoctum furfuris* for common Drink, and so much lenitive Electuary as procured her a Stool next Day. As there was a strong
Sufpicion of her having a Stone, she was founded ; but nothing
at all was to be felt in the Bladder. Her Medicines eased her
Pain in making Water, but not the Pain in her Back. On the
16th her Water was thick and turbid, and deposited a brown
Sediment ; and the Difficulty in making Water still remained;
instead of the lenitive Electuary she was ordered the Rhubarb oily
Draught to be taken every Night. On the 18th, there being no
Change in her Disorder, she had Draughts made of an Ounce
and a Half of simple Mint Water, Half a Drachm of the dulcified Spirit of Nitre, and five Drops of the *tinctura thebaica,* and
Syrup three Times a-Day; but on the 22d she complained, that since
she left off the oily Medicines, her Pain and Difficulty in making

feed, or fuch other mild mucilaginous Liquors ; and to take oily Medicines and Opiates
occafionally,

king Water had grown worfe ; fhe was therefore ordered the
faline and oily Draughts alternately, and to take the Rhubarb
oily Draught occafionally when coftive, which removed thefe
Complaints ; and they did not return while fhe remained in
the Houfe ; but on the 4th of *July*, the Day before fhe was to
have been difcharged as cured, fhe was attacked with a fharp
Pain in her Hip and Loins, and about the *os coccygis* ; which
increafed till the 9th, and extended itfelf all along the Outfide of the right Thigh ; it was moft acute about the *os coccygis*; but on examining, nothing was to be obferved externally : This Pain continued more or lefs all that Month, and till
the End of the next, and fo obftinate as not to be altered by
bleeding, and the Ufe of Liniments, Blifters, cooling Medicines, Opiates, warm Baths, and other Remedies. On the
20th of *Auguft*, a ftrengthening Plaifter was applied to her
Back, which gave immediate Relief, and fhe was difcharged
cured the 29th. She continued well till *October*, when fhe was
attacked with a violent Fever at *Hounflow*, and was brought to
the Hofpital on the 24th of that Month, and the tenth Day of
the Fever. She died the 3d of *November*. During the Courfe
of the Fever, fhe only complained once of a Difficulty of making Water.—After Death I had her Body opened, when the
only Thing particular which we could obferve, was the uri-
nary Bladder about four times the natural Size ; it feemed to
be flaccid, and in a State of Relaxation ; the Kidneys were
found, and no Signs of any Diftemper could be obferved about
the Uterus or Rectum, or near the *os coccygis.* —When fhe was

Q 4   firft

occafionally, and gentle Laxatives, to keep the Body open ; which Method of Treatment ge-nerally

firft in the Hofpital, I defired her always to examine her U-rine ; but fhe never obferved that fhe paffed any Sand, Gra-vel, or any thing of that kind.

Thomae Jacey, an elderly Man, was admitted into *St.* Ge*orge's* Hofpital the 14th of *March* 1759, for a Pain in his Back, and a Difficulty and Pain in making Water, which was often mixed with grum·us Blood ; but he had never obferved any Sand or Gravel in it. His Pulfe was quick and full, attended with Heat and Thirft ; and he was inclined to be coftive ; he was at firft blooded, and took a Dofe of laxative Mixture, and two Oun-ces of the Tincture of Rofes, four Times a-Day, and the *de-coctum malvæ* for common Drink. At firft he feemed relieved, and paffed no grumous Blood for fome Days ; but on the 26th, as he complained much of a Pain in making Water, the Tinc-ture of Rofes was changed for the oily Draughts, and he was ordered the Rhubarb oily Draught occafionally. On the 9th of *April* he fell fuddenly into a comatofe Way, and remained fo till the 12th, when he died, notwithftanding the Ufe of divers Remedies.—Upon examining his Body, both Kidneys were found in a found State ; the Inteftines covered with flight in-flammatory Spots, the Bladder of Urine quite contracted, fchirrhous, and greatly thickened ; and its internal Surface rough and eroded, with one or two black Spots on it, and fome grumous Blood lying on its Surface. The other vifcera were found.

In Ulcers of thefe Organs, the natural Balfams, mixed with foft Things, are often of great Service ; of which the follow-ing

nerally gave Relief.   Where the Patients were
plethoric, or complained of Pain, or the Diforder

ing Cafe is an Example.——*William Lumley*, a Boy nine Years
of Age, was admitted into *St. George's* Hofpital, the 6th of
September 1759, for a Pain in the Bladder, and a Difficulty in
making Water, which was always more or lefs mixed with
Matter.   At firft there was a Sufpicion of his having the
Stone; but on founding, none was to be found.   From the
Symptoms, it appeared as if there was an Ulcer in the Bladder near to its Neck; the Boy had a Cough, was very low,
and inclined to be coftive; at firft he took three Spoonfuls of
the Sperma Ceti Mixture four Times a-Day, and a Dofe of
Phyfic; but the Symptoms ftill remaining, on the 2d of *October* he was ordered to take a Scruple of the *electuarium e
fpermate ceti* three or four Times a Day, and to have the Gum-
Arabic Decoction for his common Drink.   By continuing the
Ufe of thefe Things, and taking fome opiate and laxative Medicines occafionally, he mended by flow Degrees, and all his
Symptoms went off; and he recovered his Health and Strength,
and returned Thanks for his Cure the 18th of *January* 1760.

The following Account of a remarkable Suppreffion of Urine
I had in a Letter, dated the 25th of *November* 1757, from Mr.
Pearfon, one of the Surgeons to his Majefty's Military Hofpi-
tals, who then ferved as a Mate.

James Ruffenael, aged Twenty, of a delicate Habit, was, in
the Middle of *July* laft, feized with a violent Pain in both
Kidneys, which extended along the Ureters to the Bladder, and
remained in the fame Situation for about three Weeks; during
which Period his Urine began to decreafe in Quantity, and the
voiding

order was attended with a Fever, Bleeding was
often neceſſary.

When

voiding of it was attended with acute Pain about the Neck of the
Bladder. The Secretion then totally ſtopt; he remained for upwards
of five Weeks in the Hoſpital at *Dorcheſter*, and made no Water ; at the End of which Time I firſt viſited him along with
Mr. *Adair*. He complained then of a ſlight Pain in his Kidneys, and told us he had a tolerable Appetite, ſweated little,
and voided every Day four or five Liquid Stools. He was ordered Boluſes of Camphor, and *ſal. vol. c. cervi*, and every
Night a Doſe of *tinctura cantharidum*; which he continued to
take for a Fortnight without receiving the leaſt Benefit. I
then blooded him to the Quantity of ten Ounces, and gave
him an Emetic of ſix Drachms of the *vinum ipecacoanhæ*, and
two Ounces of the Oxymel of Squills, which operated very
well ; and afterwards ordered him to take one of the following
Boluſes every four Hours. ℞ Sapon. dur. Hiſpan. drachm. i.
Sal. Abſynth. gr. vi. Calc. Viv. gr. x. Balſam. Peruv. q. s.
ut fiat Bolus. Theſe he continued to take for twelve Days.
On the Morning of the 14th of *October*, he was ſuddenly ſeized with an acute Pain in both Kidneys, and about Noon
voided upwards of Half a Pint of ſtraw-coloured Urine, which
let fall a clay-coloured Sediment. As he was feveriſh, I took
away twelve Ounces of Blood, and ordered him Barley Water
with Nitre for Drink. He was eaſy in the Night, and made
upwards of two Pints of Urine, which depoſited a Sediment of
a gelatinous Conſiſtence. Next Morning the Pain increaſed,
eſpecially in his Right Side, and ten Ounces more of Blood
was taken away : This lowered the Pulſe, and conſiderably

abated

When the Stoppage, of Urine feemed to arife from an Inflammation of the Kidneys or Bladder, or other Difeafes of thefe Parts, we

abated the Pain. Both this and the Blood taken away the Day before threw up an inflammatory Buff. He was ordered to continue the Ufe of the Barley Water with Nitre, and to take three Spoonfuls of a Mixture with *fpiritus mindereri* every two Hours. He had an eafy Night, and was next Day free from Fever ; but complained of an Uneafinefs in his Stomach and Naufea. He was ordered a Scruple of the Powder of Ipecacoanha, which vomited him, and procured him a Stool. He was eafy in the Night ; but in the Morning was hot, and complained of a Pain in his Right Kidney, and all over his Bones, as he exprefled it. I then gave him a Mixture, with *fpiritus mindereri*, and the *pulvis contrayerva comp.* of which I defired him to take fome Spoonfuls frequently. This procured him a plentiful Sweat, which removed the Fever and Pain: thefe Symptoms returned next Day, but were removed by the fame Means. I remained at *Dorchefter* for a Week after, and he recovered his Strength and Appetite as much as could be expeeted in fo fhort a Time ; but he ftill complained of Pain in his Right Kidney, tho' he made Water freely. By a Letter I received from the Gentleman whofe Care I left him under, I un-underftood he had a Relapfe, which he has fince got the bet-ter of.   .

I forgot to inform you, that his Father died of the fame Complaints, after being fix Months without fecreting a Drop of Urine ; and his Brother died of the fame in about ten Weeks.

treated

treated it accordingly; and where the Fever was confiderable, we made Evacuations, and gave plenty of diluting Liquors, and the cooling faline Medicines, and afterwards thofe of the foft, mucilaginous, and oily Nature, and mild Diuretics and Opiates.

When the Diforder, in its Progrefs, became chronical, the Sick were commonly fent down to the fixed Hofpital, fo that we had no Opportunity of examining the Bodies of fuch as might die of this Complaint.

O F

OF THE

EPILEPSY.

THE Epilepſy, or Falling Sickneſs, attacked a Number of Men, from the
ſevere Duty of long Marches in hot Weather,
and afterwards lying out on the cold Ground,
expoſed to the Damps of the Night (*a*).
It was very ſeldom that Men were cured of
this Diſorder in the military Hoſpitals. We
had ſome few Inſtances, indeed, where Relief ſeemed to be obtained by Reſt, a regular

- (*a*) I ſaw above twenty Men, while I was in *German.*, who
attributed the Epileptic Fits they were attacked with to theſe
Cauſes, and ſaid they had never had the Epilepſy before ; beſides others, who had been formerly ſubjeſt to theſe Fits, who
declared, that the Diſorder was brought back by the ſante
Means.

Diet,

Diet, gentle Evacuations, and Iſſues (*b*) ; but
even thoſe Men generally relapſed as ſoon as
they

(*b*) *William Wilſon*, a Boy fourteen Years of Age, was admitted into *St. George*'s Hoſpital, *Sept.* 20, 1758, for Epileptic
Fits, which he had been ſubject to for ſome Time, and which
generally ſeized him three or four Times a Week.   He took
Variety of Medicines without any Effect till the 6th of *November*, when I ordered him to take eight Grains of the *pilulæ fœ-
tidæ* Morning and Evening, and Phyſic twice a Week, and a
Seton to be made in his Neck.   After the Seton began to run,
he had but three or four ſlight Fits in *November*, and none the
following Month ; and he was diſcharged the Hoſpital the 3d
of *January* 1759, ſeemingly in good Health, with Directions to
keep the Seton running at leaſt for ſome Months after he went
home, and to come again to the Hoſpital if he ſhould have any
Return of his Fits ; but we never heard more of him.

Mary Hacket, a Girl of nineteen Years of Age, was admitted
into *St. George*'s Hoſpital the 14th of *February* 1759, for Fits.
The Account ſhe gave of her Caſe, was, that about five Years
before ſhe was ſeized with the firſt Fit, after a Fright ; three
Years afterwards ſhe had a ſecond Fit, and for ſome Time after
had a Fit commonly once a Month, about the Time of the
full Moon ; and ſince had them more frequently ; that the Fits
began with a Trembling and Shaking of the right Foot, and
ſhe had frequent pricking Pains in the right Thigh, and what
ſhe called convulſive Tremors in the right Leg and Foot.   She
was regular in her menſtrual Diſcharge.   At the Time ſhe
came into the Hoſpital, ſhe was feveriſh, and complained much
of a ſharp Pain in the right Thigh : She was blooded, and took
ſome

they were fent to their Regiments, and began to do Duty. All who had thefe Fits after being fome Time with their Regiments, were at laft difcharged, and fent home. However, before Men are difcharged for Fits, they fhould be watched very narrowly for fome Time; for there is no Diforder which Soldiers are more apt to counterfeit than this.

It is no Wonder that Soldiers, during the Time of Service, fhould feldom be cured of thefe Fits; for in Adults it is not often cured

fome cooling Medicine, and had no Fit till the 9th of *March*: She then took the fetid Pills and camphorated Julep twice a Day; but ftill the Fits returned frequently. She then had the Bark, Valerian and Purging Dofes fucceffively, and ufed the warm Bath; but without any Effect. On the 7th of *May* a Blifter was applied to her right Foot, which was intended to be kept open; but an Inflammation coming on that Leg and Foot, it was fuffered to dry up, and an Iffue made in the fame Leg. From the Time the Blifter was applied, fhe had no Fit while fhe remained in the Hofpital. She was difcharged the 15th of *July*, feemingly in good Health; though during that Period fhe had fome little Tremors in her Foot, and was fub-ject to be low and faintifh, which was always relieved by cordial anodyne Medicines. After going out of the Hofpital, fhe remained in good Health for feven or eight Months, when I was told her Difeafe had returned as violent as ever.

even

even in private Practice, with all the Conveniencies and Advantages to be wifhed
for; and generally the few that do get well,
require a confiderable Length of Time to ac-
complifh the Cure; and we find from daily
Experience, as well as from examining the
Records of Medicine, that the Cures that have
been made, have moftly been performed either
by a Change of Air, fuch as going from a cold
to a hot Climate (*c*), by fome remarkable
Change of Life (*d*), or fome accidental Diforder;

(*c*) *Hippocrates* lays the chief Strefs of the Cure upon Change
of Air, Aphor. 4, 5, fect. ii. The Baron *Van Sweiten* fays, he has
known a great Number cured by going to the *Eaft Indies*; many of
whom have remained well ever after, while others had a Return
of the Diforder when they came back to *Holland*. *Comment.*
vol. III. p. 436. fect. 1080.

(*d*) *Celfus* has long ago obferved, that the Appearance of the
Menfes in Girls, and of Puberty in Boys, often removes this
Diforder, lib. iii. cap. xxiii.—On the 22d of *November* 1758,
Mary Evans, a Girl of eighteen Years of Age, was admitted
into *St. George*'s Hofpital for Fits. She had never had the
Menftrua; but, for above two Years, found regularly, once a
Month, a Fulnefs in her Breafts, and had a flight Head Ach,
and other Symptoms which generally precede this Difcharge;
and were fucceeded with violent Epileptic Fits, which continu-
ed

der (*e*) ; or by Iffues or Drains (*f*) ; or by the
Removal of fome acrid or irritating Subftance,

ed returning frequently for two or three Days, and then went
off; and fhe had no more Symptoms of them, till about the
fame Time next Month. She was ordered to take ten Grains
of the *pilulæ fætidæ* Morning and Evening, and a Dofe of Phyfic twice a Week; and as I found that fhe became plethoric
near the Time her Fits ufed to return, I began to imagine, that
both the Fits and Stoppage of the Menftrua were owing to too
great a Fullnefs of the Veffels, which prevented the Heart and
vafcular Syftem from having fuch free Play, as to drive the
Blood through the extreme uterine Veffels : I therefore ordered
feven Ounces of Blood to be taken away from her immediately.
In three Days Time the menftrual Difcharge began to make its
Appearance; and on the 10th of *January* fhe was difcharged
the Hofpital, feemingly in good Health, after the menftrual
Difcharge had returned for two regular Periods, without any
Appearance of Epileptic Fits. She was defired to come back
to the Hofpital, if the Fits returned; but I never heard more
of her.

(*e*) *William Glen*, a Patient in the *Royal Infirmary* at *Edinburgh*
in *September* 1747, was freed from Epileptic Fits, which ufed to
return ten or twelve Times a Day, for a Quarter of a Year, by
a Diarrhœa coming on; but they afterwards returned.

A Man fubject to the Epilepfy was cured of it by a Quartan
Ague, and had afterwards no Return of the Diforder. *Mifcell.
Curiof. Dec.* 3. *Ann.* 3. p. 34.

(*f*) There are numerous Inftances of the good Effects of
Iffues and Drains in diverfe Authors. *Tulpius, Van Swieten,
&c.*

R   or

or fuch like (*g*) ; or by preventing the
Caufe (*h*) ; and that thofe Medicines called
Specifics have in general had but little Share in
the Cure.

(*g*) *La Motte* gives one Inftance of a Perfon being cured of
the Epilepfy by voiding five Stones, *Chirurg.* vol. II. p. 20 ;
and of another who died of the Fits from a triangular Stone
remaining in the Kidneys, *ibid.* p. 416.   Dr. *Short* cured a Woman of an Epilepfy of twelve Years ftanding, by extirpating a
cartilagenous Subftance, about the Bignefs of a large Pea, feated on the gaftronemei Mufcles, above a Nerve which he cut
afunder.   *Edin. Medic. Effays,* vol. IV. Art. 27.

(*h*) *Galen,* tells us, of his having prevented the Epileptic Fits
in a Boy, who ufed to have one whenever he was hungry, by
making him carry Bread in his Pocket, and eat a little as foon
as he found the leaft Symptoms of Hunger.   *De Loc. Affect.*
lib. v. cap. vi.——And *Van Sweiten* mentions how he cured a
Boy, who had a Fit every full Moon ; whofe under Lip ufed to
fall a Trembling before it began (a Symptom which, he fays,
often precedes Vomiting) ; by giving a Vomit every Month,
for fix Months fucceffively, three Days before the full Moon,
and an Opiate in the Evening after its Operation ; and by putting him under a Courfe of ftrengthening Medicines.   It was
obferveable, that if he vomited in the Time of the Paroxyfm,
it was foon at an End.   See his *Comment.* vol. III. p. 439. fect.
1050.

O F

OF THE

SMALL - POX.

THE Small Pox appeared at *Paderborn* in the Spring 1761, and five had the diftinct Kind, who recovered. Six or feven had them at *Ofnabruck* in *May* and *June*, and one Man and a Child died of the confluent Kind. Four had the diftinct Kind at *Munfter* in *July* and *Auguft*, who all did well. During the Winter, we had fixteen in the Hofpital I attended at *Bremen*; ten had the diftinct Kind, and all recovered; five had the confluent Kind, of whom two died; as did alfo one who was brought to the Hofpital with all the Symptoms of the moft malignant Kind. Two were fent to *Natzungen* in *July*, both ill of the confluent Kind; the one died two Hours after his Arri-

val;

val; the other recovered: And we had only two in the Hofpital at *Ofnabruck* in Winter 1762-63, and both did well.

There was nothing particular either in the Courfe or Treatment of this Diforder, different from what we meet with in daily Practice; only as the Soldiers, who were attacked with it, were ftrong, and in full Health, they required Bleeding and gentle Evacuations, and a cooling Regimen, on the firft Appearance of the Symptoms.

The malignant Kind required the Ufe of Acids, and the Bark; which laft, could often only be adminiftered by Way of Clyfter, as the Sick could not fwallow it: In fhort, we treated the Patients much in the fame Way as in the malignant Fever, Allowance only being made for the prefent Circumftances.

Luckily this Diforder never fpread much in the Army, while I was in *Germany*.

O F

O F

Erisypilatous Swellings.

IN *January* 1762, feveral Patients in the
Hofpitals I had the Care of at *Bremen*,
had fhining watery Swellings of the Face, or
Extremities; which came fuddenly, and were
attended with a flight Degree of Inflammation, and watery Blifters rifing above the Skin,
and fome Degree of Fever. The Blifters were
not fmall, round, and angry, as in *St. Antony's*
Fire; but larger, and of an irregular Figure,
refembling thofe raifed when People are fcalded
by boiling Water. The Swellings did not pit
on being preffed, as the eodematous Swellings
commonly do : They gave Pain when preffed,
but the Inflammation was not in that high
Degree as it is in the common Phlegmon :

The

The Blood was fizy, and the Water of a high Colour. The Diforder feemed to be a Species of the Erifypelas.

Between the 9th and 12th of *January*, three Patients were feized with fuch Swellings.

The firft was a Dragoon, who had juft recovered from a Flux, and a bad Cough. On the 9th, he was fuddenly feized in the Night with a large Swelling of his Face, Hands, and Arms, which had a fhining oedemetous Appearance, with a fmall Degree of Rednefs, and was painful when preffed; and he had two or three watery Blifters rofe on the Back of each Hand above the Divifion of the Fingers, attended with a quick full Pulfe, a feverifh Heat and Thirft, a Cough, and fomewhat of a Difficulty of Breathing, and high-coloured Water; and he was inclined to be coftive. He was immediately blooded, had a faline Mixture with Contrayerva and Nitre, and was ordered to take a Purge in the Morning. Next Day the Blood had thrown up an infl-mmatory Buff, the Fever was abated, and the Breathing eafier; but the Cough and Swelling ftill remained.

mained. He then took a Julep made of equal
Parts of the Saline and Sperma Ceti Mixtures,
which eaſed the Cough. The fourth Day the
Pulſe was ſoft, and the Swellings ſtill in the
ſame Situation, and the Breathing a little affected. A large Bliſter was applied to his Back,
which diſcharged plentifully, relieved the
Breathing, and leſſened the Swellings conſiderably. The Cough and ſome Degree of
Swelling ſtill remained; but were removed
by the Uſe of the Sperma Ceti Mixture with
Oxymel, gentle Opiates, and ſome Doſes of
Phyſic.

The ſecond was a Man of the Twentieth
Regiment of Foot, who had been ſome
Months in the Hoſpital for a hectic Complaint;
he was taken ill, the ſame Night as the
Dragoon, with a Swelling of his whole Face,
particularly the Lips, which had a ſhining watery Appearance, and a ſlight Degree of Redneſs, attended with a ſtrong Fever; and was
cured by Bleeding, Purging, the Uſe of the
ſaline Medicines, and the Application of a
Bliſter.

R 4 The

The third was an Invalid, who had been admitted for a pleuritic Complaint, which he had got the better of. He was attacked, the second Night after the other two, with a ſhineing, watery, reddiſh Swelling, of his right Hand and Arm, up as far as the Joint of the Shoulder; four large watery Bladders likewiſe appeared on the fore Part of his Arm, above the Joint of the Elbow. Bleeding, with the cooling Medicines, and two Doſes of Salts, carried off the Fever, and leſſened the Swelling, in about ſeven Days Time; but a little of it, with a Stiffneſs, ſtill remained; which at laſt was removed by the Uſe of aromatic Fomentations, rubbing with the *linimentum ſaponaceum*, and taking two Doſes of Phyſic.

Within leſs than a Fortnight, five or ſix more were ſeized with Swellings of the ſame Kind on ſome of the Extremities, and all got well by nearly the ſame Treatment; excepting one Man, who was in a very low State, and had a large deep Ulcer on his Hip, where there had been a Mortification from his lying on that Part in a Fever. The Swelling at firſt

feemed

feemed to give Way; but on the third or fourth Day, having got a fevere Cough, the Swelling increafed, and the Inflammation began to look livid, and the Difcharge from the Sore to look bad; and, notwithftanding various Means were ufed, a Mortification of the Part came on, and he died the feventh Day.

O F

S C U R V Y.

THE true Scurvy, attended with fpungy fetid Gums of a livid Colour, with livid Blotches, and Ulcers of the Legs, and other Symptoms, began to fhew itfelf at *Bremen* in *Ja-nuary* 1762 ; tho' we had not the leaft Appear-ance of this Diforder in the Hofpitals at any other Place, while I was with the Troops in *Germany*.

A great Variety of Diforders have been call-. ed by the Name of Scurvy: and the Difeafe has been divided into hot and cold ; into the Acid, the Alcaline; and the Muriatic, according to the different Fancies of Authors, and the Caufes they imagined it took its Rife from ; but, from later and more acurate Obfervations, Dr. *Lind* has

has juftly remarked, that the true Scurvy has
been found to be the fame in all the different
Parts of the Globe, and to take its Rife from
fimilar Caufes ; from Cold and Moifture, and
living much upon falted Provifions, joined to
a Want of frefh Vegetables, and of good generous fermented Liquors; and hence it is moft
frequent in low marfhy Places in northern Climates, where there is a Scarcity of frefh Vegi-
tables ; and where the Inhabitants live much
upon falted Provifions in Winter; and aboard of
Ships in long Voyages or Cruizes, efpecially in
the northern Seas : and hence this Diforder
was fo frequent at *Quebec* the firft Winter it was
in our Poffeffion; and in fome of the other Forts
in *North America*, which were taken fo late in
the Year, that the Troops had not fufficient
Time to lay in a Stock of Vegetables, and of
frefh Meat to be preferved by the Froft (*a*) ; but
were obliged to live moftly on Ship Provifions.

It

(*a*) In *Quebec*, and other northern Parts of *North America*, as
foon as the Froft fets in, they kill their Meat intended for their
Winter

It is obferved, both at Sea and Land, that where the Scurvy rages, thofe People are leaft fubject to it who are well cloathed ; who live in dry Habitations, or lie in dry Births ; who take proper Exercife, without being too much expofed to the Inclemency of the Weather ; and who live well, and drink good Beer, Cyder, or Wine ; as has been remarked by Dr. *Pringle*, Dr. *Lind*, and others.

At *Bremen* the Diforder was only obferved among the Soldiers ; not one of the Gentlemen belonging to the Hofpital, or to the Commiffariate, nor one of the military Officers, not even of the Serjeants, having the leaft Symptom of it. The Reafon of its being frequent among the Soldiers was, that the Place is fituated on a Plain naturally very damp ; and the Soldiers were quartered in very low damp Houfes ; at the fame Time, no Vegetables or

Winter Store, and hang it up : It foon freezes, and will keep in this Manner all through the Winter. They preferve Vegetables in the fame Way ; and when they intend to make Ufe of either, they put fo much as they want into cold Water for fome Time, which draws the Froft out of it ; and then they boil or roaft it, as they think proper.

Greens

Greens were to be bought in the Market; and frefh Meat, and other frefh Provifions, were at fo high a Price, that the Soldiers could not afford to buy them; but were obliged to live on falted Meat, and falted Herrings, during the Winter; and what little Money they had remaining, they laid out on fpirituous Liquors, which were fold cheap.

The Cure of this Diforder requires—living in a dry comfortable Place—good Cloathing—light Food of eafy Digeftion, fuch as good Bread, Panado, Milk, Whey, Broths made of frefh Meats—white Meats, with Greens, or other Vegetable, &c.—the Ufe of Liquors of the acid or acefcent Kind, or the moderate Ufe of Beer, Cyder, good Wine, or weak Punch (*b*) —And, by Way of Medicine, gentle Purges, mild Diaphoretics; the free Ufe of acid or acefcent Fruits, Lemons, Oranges, Apples, Pears,

(*b*) The free Ufe of raw Spirits is found to be very prejudicial; but a moderate Quantity of thefe Spirits, diluted with Water, and acidulated with Lemons or Oranges (or with Cream of Tartar, or Tamarinds, when the former cannot be got), and made into Punch, is found to be a good Antifcorbutic.

Currans,

Currans, Grapes, &c. and of the antifcorbutic
Plants and their Juices, as Succory, Endive,
Water-Crefles, Scurvy-Grafs (c), &c. on which
a great Part of the Cure principally depends;
and the Ufe of fome of the ftrengthening Bitters (d), of which the Bark is not the leaft efficacious.

Bleeding is feldom requifite, except where
there is much Heat or Fever; or a fharp Pain

(c) Moft ripe Fruits, particularly Lemons and Oranges, and
efculent Herbs, and many Kinds of Roots, fuch as Horfe-Radifh, Onions, Leeks, and many others, have been found the moft
ufeful Remedies in the Cure of the Scurvy. Decoctions and
Infufions of Fir-Tops, of Spruce, and of other Species of the
Pine-Tree; and Beer made of thefe Infufions, by fermenting
them with Molaffes, are approved Antifcorbutics: and when
fuch Remedies cannot be got, Infufions of the common Bitters,
and weak Punch, made with Tamarinds or Cream of Tartar,
have proved ferviceable; and where thefe Acids cannot be had,
the Mineral Acids may be ufed for aciduiating the Drink.
However, it ought always to be remembered, that frefh Vegetables and Fruits, and vegitable Acids, produce much better
Effects in the Scurvy, than any other Sorts of Remedies; and
ought always to be ufed, when they can be got.

(d) Moft of the common Bitters have been ftrongly recommended in this Diforder, Gentian, Trifoil, Wormwood, &c.—
as likewife aromatic Bitters and Aromatics; fuch as *calamus
aromaticus,* Carvi Seeds, Winters Bark, Cinamon, and many
others.

of

of the Side, or Difficulty of Breathing, or fome
Symptom of the like Kind ; it is then fometimes neceffary to take away fome Blood : And
in obftinate Cafes, it is often found of Ufe to
promote Sweats, by making the Patient, while
in Bed, drink freely of warm Whey, or Sack
Whey, mixed with the fcorbutic Juices ; or
warm Barley Water, or the like, mixed with a
fmall Quantity of the Antimonial Wine, or fome
other mild Diaphoretic.

And where the Patient is ftrong, and there
is no Danger of Hœmorrhagies, warm aromatic Baths have fometimes been found ferviceab-
ab!e ; but they are not to be ufed where the
Patient is weak.

The firft Time I faw this Diforder at *Bremen*, was in an old Invalid, *James Long*, who
had come from *Briftol* to *Embden*, and from
thence to *Bremen*. He was fome Weeks in the
Hofpital before I difcovered his Diforder to be
the Scurvy. He at firft complained only of
great Weaknefs, and fuch a Giddinefs, when
he got out of Bed, that he could not walk, and
of what he called flying rheumatic Pains of his
Legs.

Legs.   He had no other vifible Complaint; all
which, I imagined, proceeded from Old-Age,
and being worn out in the Service.   At laft,
on the 25th of *January*, he complained of his
Gums being fore ; and, on examining him, I
found his Breath fetid, his Gums fwelled, foft,
and fpungy, his Legs covered with fcorbutic
Blotches, and other Symptoms, which evidently proved his Diforder to be the true
Scurvy.

Upon which, I ordered him a low Diet, with
the Addition of Greens for Dinner, and a Quart
of Lemonade, with a Gill of Brandy in it, *per*
Day, for his common Drink ; and, by Way of
Medicine, a Decoction of the Bark, with the
Elixir of Vitriol ; and, at the fame Time, ordered his Gums to be fcarified, where they
were moft fwelled and fpungy ; and to be
wafhed frequently with an aftringent Gargle ;
and to be rubbed now and then with burnt
Alum (*e*).   By thefe Means, in a Fortnight's
Time

(*e*) Dr. *Lind*, who has wrote one of the beft Treatifes on this
Diforder, and who had a great Deal of Practice himfelf, fays,
" When

Time, his Gums became firmer, and his fcorbutic Symptoms decreafed. During that Courfe
he took cold, and had a Stitch in his Side, for
which he was blooded. The Blood threw up
a very thin Buff, which was not of a firm Confiftence (*f*); the Craffamentum below was of
a blackifh

" When firft the Patient complains of an Itching and a Spun-
" ginefs of the Gums, with loofe Teeth, either a Tincture of
" the Bark in Brandy, or aluminous Medicines, will be found
" ferviceable in putting a Stop to the Beginning Laxity of
" thefe Parts." When the Putrefaction increafes; he recommends the Ufe of fome of the mineral Acids. See his *Treatife
en the Scurvy*, part ii. chap. v. p. 201.—*Van Swieten* fays, he
never found any Thing anfwer better than a Gargle made of
four Ounces of Elder or Rofe Water, acidulated with a Drachm
of the Spirit of Sea Salt ; and where the Gums were very putrid and gangrened, he has been obliged to touch them flightly
with the pure Acid Spirit, and fome Hours after to have them
wafhed with the Gargle juft mentioned. Vide *Comment.* vol. III.
p. 629, fect. 1163.

If the Spunginefs of the Gums fprout out into a luxuriant
Fungus, it is fometimes requifite to cut fuch Fungufes away,
and to wafh the Sores frequently with gentle aftringent or acid
Liquors.

Dr. *Huxham* obferves, that, after the Difeafe has continued
fome Time, the Blood appears a mere Gore as it were, not fe-
parating into Serum and Craffamentum as ufual, but remaining
an uniform half-coagulated Mafs, generally of a more livid or

a blackifh Colour and of a loofe Texture, and
the Serum in a large Proportion. By the 2d
of *March* his Gums had recovered their natural Firmnefs and Texture, and the fcorbutic
Spots and Pains of the Legs were gone, and he
had recovered his Strength; the only remaining Complaint was a little Swelling about the
Ankles, for which he continued the fame
Courfe, and took a Dofe or two of Phyfic.
By the 16th of *March* all thefe Symptoms
were gone, and he was difmiffed the Hofpital
free from all Complaints. I faw him well the
laft Week in *May*; and he told me, he had
had no fcorbutic Symptom fince he left the
Hofpital.

darker Colour than common; though fometimes it continues
long very florid; but it always putrifies foon. See his *Effay on
Fevers*, chap. v.

There is fomething very particular in the Nature of this
Diforder, according to an Obfervation of Dr. *Lind*'s; who
fays, " That the Scurvy is a Difeafe in its Nature very oppo-
" fite to that of a Fever; infomuch, that even an Infection
" is long refifted by a fcorbutic Habit; and thofe of a fcorbu-
" tic Habit being feized with the Fever, was a Proof of its
" proceeding entirely from Infection." See his *Firft Paper on
Fevers*, p. 4.

In

In the Beginning of *February*, another of the Invalids, who had been in the Hofpital for a Fever and rheumatic Complaints, had Blotches appeared on his Legs, complained of great Weaknefs, and fainted away in attempting to walk; which made me fufpect his Diforder to be the Scurvy; and, on examining him, I found his Gums foft and fpongy, attended with the other Symptoms of the true Scurvy. I put him nearly on the fame Courfe as in the laft-mentioned Cafe : He ufed a low Diet, with the Addition of Greens for Dinner, which he eat with a little Butter and Vinegar ; and he had a Quart of Lemonade, with two Ounces of Brandy, for his common Drink during the Day; and, by Way of Medicine, a Decoction of the Bark, with two Drachms of the *confectio cordiaca* to each Half Pint, which he took by Spoonfuls. Next Day he complained of a Pain in his Leg; and, on examining it more particularly, I found a large livid Blotch, yellow all round the Edges, on the fore Part, and a Tenfion all over that Leg. As he was fo extremely low, as to be in Danger of

S 2   fainting

fainting whenever he fat up, I was afraid left a Mortification fhould enfue; and therefore ordered his Leg to be bathed Morning and Evening with a warm aromatic Fomentation, and a Poultice of Theriaca to be applied after it; and defired him to take as much of the Decoction of the Bark with the Cordial as pof-fible; and allowed him a Glafs of Mountain Wine every two or three Hours. By the Continuance of this Courfe for fome Weeks, the livid Blotches, Pain, and Stiffnefs of his Leg, and moft of the other fcorbutic Symp-toms, went away; his Gums were reftored to their natural Firmnefs; and he recovered his Strength fo much as to be able to fit up all Day long; though he ftill remained very weak when he was fent to *England*, in *March*.

In *February* and *March*, feven or eight more fcorbutic Patients were fent to the Hofpital I attended, who were all treated in the famo Manner; and all did well. About the Middle of *February* this Diftemper began to fhew it-felf in the other Hofpital attended by Dr. *Miller*,

who

who treated the Patients nearly in the fame
Way, and they all recovered.

On the 5th of *April,* a young Man, belonging to the Eighth Regiment of Foot, came to
the Hofpital with all the Symptoms of the true
Scurvy ; his Gums were fpungy and fœtid ; he
had livid Blotches on his Legs, and Contrac-
tions of the Hams, and a Stiffnefs and Hardnefs in the Calves of both Legs (*g*). By following the fame Courfe as the others, and the
Ufe of frequent Fomentations, and rubbing the
contracted Parts with foft Liniments, he mended daily ; and, after taking a Dofe or two of
Phyfic, was difmiffed perfectly recovered on
the 10th of *May.* At his firft Admiffion into
the Hofpital, he was taken with a fevere Cough,

(*g*) If the Swellings became large, ftiff, and painful, Dr.
Lind recommends that the Legs fhould be frequently bathed
and fomented ; or, what he has found preferable, to be expofed to their Steams, after being well covered with Blankets.
After this Operation, he advifes the Limb to be rubbed with
fome mild Oil, fuch as *oleum palmæ,* or Salad Oil ; and if the
Swellings refift both the general Cure and thefe Applications,
the Limbs to be fweated with Spirits. See his *Treatife on the
Scurvy,* part ii. chap. v.

attended

attended with Pain of the Breaft, and a Spitting of Blood for a Day or two, for which he
was blooded. His Blood threw up a little
Buff; the Craffamentum was of a blackifh Colour and of a loofe Texture, with a good Proportion of a yellowifh Serum. This Bleeding
relieved the Complaints of his Breaft, and he
had no Return of them while he remained in
the Hofpital.

The firft Week in *May* four Invalids were
admitted into the Hofpital for this Diforder.
The firft had fpungy Gums, a fœtid Breath,
his Legs fwelled and hard, and of a deep pur-
ple Colour. The fecond was a Cafe at firft of
a more doubtful Kind; there were no fpungy
Gums, though an offenfive Breath; his Ancles
and Feet were fwelled, attended with Pain and
Uneafinefs, and a great Weaknefs and Laffi-
tude; but no Fever, nor any livid Blotches.
The Swelling of the Feet and Ancles feemed
at firft Sight rather gouty or rheumatic, than of
the fcorbutic Kind; but from the Man's Way
of Life, and the Diforder being fo frequent, we
difcovered it to be the Scurvy. The third had
a very

a very fœtid Breath and fpungy Gums, livid
Spots and fungous Ulcers (*h*) on his Legs, with
Pains and Weaknefs all over. The fourth had
alfo fpungy Gums and a fœtid Breath, Pains of
the Legs and Arms, livid Blotches on his Legs,
great Hardnefs and Contraction of the right
Ham, and a livid hard Swelling on the Outfide
of the left Thigh, immediately above the
Knee.

We treated them all four in the Method
above-mentioned, adding a Mefs of Greens to

(*h*) " Ulcers on the Legs, or any other Part of the Body,
" require pretty much the fame Treatment, *viz.* very gentle
" Compreffion, in order to keep under the Fungus, and fuch
" antifceptic Applications as have been recommended for pu-
" trid Gums, *viz. mel refat.* acidulated with *fpiritus vitrioli,*
" *ung. Ægiptiacum, &c.* but nothing will avail where the Pa-
" tient cannot have Vegetables and Fruits." *Dr. Lind's Treatife on Scurvy,* part ii. chap. v. p. 204. And he recommends,
if the Swellings and Ulcers of the Legs neither yield to the general Cure nor to the Methods here propofed, that a flow and
gentle Courfe of Mercury fhould be tried, after the fcorbutic
Taint is a good deal removed, and the Gums are fufficiently
firm; and to give along with it a Decoction of the Woods, or
of Sarfapariila; but this Method ought not to be attempted till
the Gums have acquired a proper Firmnefs. See *ibid.* part ii.
chap. v.

S 4 Dinner,

Dinner, giving Lemonade for Drink, and the
Bark, with Elixir of Vitriol, by Way of Medicine. The Parts that were hard and fwelled,
were fomented, and rubbed with foft Liniments, and Poultices were applied to the hard
Swelling on the Outfide of the left Thigh; and
the Ulcers of the Legs dreffed with Digeftives,
and occafionally wafhed with fpirituous Tinc-
tures, and touched with Efcharotics. Before
I left *Bremen*, the firft Week in *June*, the firft
and fecond Patients were perfectly recovered,
and the third and fourth almoft well. All of
them had had the Diforder fome Months before they came to the Hofpital.

O F

OF THE

I T C H.

THERE was no Diforder fo common in
the military Hofpitals as the Itch. It
is of an infectious Nature, and now moft commonly believed to be entirely owing to little
Infects lodged in the Skin, which many Authors affirm they have feen in the Puftules by
the Help of a Microfcope ; and that the Diforder is entirely communicated by Infection, and
does not arife from any Fault in the Fluids or
Solids.

It has been found by Experience, that internal Medicines have little or no Effect in removing this Diforder ; and that only external
Remedies, which come immediately in contact
with the Parts affected, are capable of making a
Cure ;

Cure ; which has been brought as a farther Proof, that the Itch is owing to Animalcules or Infects ; as it is alledged, that no Remedies will cure the Diftemper, but fuch as are capable of killing them.

The-Medicines, which are moft commonly ufed for the Cure, are *Mercury, White Hele-bore,* and *Sulphur.*

Mercurial Frictions on the Part are often made ufe of, and fometimes with Succefs, though they are by no Means to be depended upon for a Cure ; befides that, they are liable to throw the Patients into a Salivation, as I have feen happen more than once ; for which Reafons I would never recommend this Method where the Patient labours under no other Diforder which requires the Ufe of Mercury, and would confine it entirely to Cafes where Patients, having the Itch, labour, at the fame Time, under the *Lues venerea,* and require the free Ufe of mercurial Frictions ; under fuch Circumftances the mercurial Ointment may be as well rubbed on the Parts affected with the Itch as upon any other.

The

The Powder of the Root of *White Helebore*, made up into an Ointment with Hogs Lard, or a strong Decoction of it in Water, rubbed on the Parts, will often cure the Itch ; but it is a sharp Medicine, and generally smarts, and sometimes inflames the Parts on which it is rubbed ; and therefore it is not so commonly used, as we know a much surer and milder Remedy. Though I have cured some People with the Helebore Lotion without any Inconvenience, who would not use the Sulphur on Account of its Smell.

Sulphur is the most certain and easy Cure for the Itch of any we know, and perhaps is more certain in the Cure of this Disorder than almost any other Medicine in any other Disorder whatever. We used it in Form of the Sulphur Ointment of the *London Dispensatory*, of which one, two, or more Drachms were rubbed in every Night, in Proportion to the Extent of the Parts affected. These Unctions were continued from four or five to ten or twelve Nights, according to the Violence and Continuance of the Disorder. Most were cured

in

in a few Days; others required a longer Time. As the fulphureous Unctions tend to obftruct the Perfpiration, we generally ordered a Purge to be given before rubbing the Sulphur Ointment, and in full Habits fometimes ordered a little Blood to be taken away; and put them all under a low Diet. After the Diforder feemed to be removed, they took another Dofe or two of Phyfic to carry off any Impurities that might have been thrown upon the Bowels, during the Ufe of the Sulphur Ointment. In inveterate Cafes, the Sulphur was given internally at the fame Time that the Patient rubbed with the Ointment.

It is generally believed (though denied by fome) that Sulphur, taken internally, enters the Blood; and its Steams are thrown off by the perfpiratory Veffels, and affifts more effectually to deftroy the Infects and their Ovula, which give Rife to the Itch; but whether this Effect be true or not, I found it to anfwer another very good Purpofe; which was to keep the Belly rather loofe, while the Patient ufed the Unction; and by this Way it carried off thofe

Humours,

Humours, which ought to have paffed off by
the Skin ; and for that Reafon, when it had
not that Effect, we joined fome Lenitive Electuary to it.

There is one Thing to be obferved with
regard to fulphureous Unctions, which is, that
we ought not to ufe them too foon with People recovering out of Fevers, or other Diforders which bring them low; otherwife there
will be Danger of bringing on a Relapfe, which
I have often obferved to happen in military
Hofpitals, where the Itch has appeared as the
Patients were recovering from Fevers and other
Diforders, and the Unctions were ufed too
foon : But whether thefe Relapfes were owing
to the fulphureous Unction's flopping up the
Pores of the Skin, and obftructing a free Perfpiration, or to the Patient's being more apt to
take Cold while they ufed the Sulphur Ointment, than at any other Time, is what I cannot determine ; but to me it feems moft pro-
bable, that thefe Unctions rather obftruct the
Perfpiration ; and that when they are ufed too
foon with People recovering from Fevers, efpecially

pecially thofe of the putrid Kind, they preveñ̃
thofe Particles from paffing off by the Skin;
which it was neceffary fhould be evacuated, in
order to free the Body from the Seeds of the
Fever, or other Diforders the Patients laboured
under. But however this be, Experience has
fhewn, that we ought not to attempt the Cure
of the Itch, in Patients fo circumftanced, till
their Strength be in a great Meafure re-efta-
blifhed, otherwife there will be Danger of a
Relapfe; and likewife, that Patients ufing Sulphur externally, ought to be particularly on
their Guard againft Cold.

This Obfervation of Peoples being fo apt to
relapfe after Fevers by the too early Ufe of fulphureous Unction, is a ftrong Proof of the Ufe-
fulnefs of keeping the Body open during the
Time of Rubbing and of Purging the Patient
afterwards; as by thefe Means we may carry
off by the Bowels thofe Particles which could
not pafs by the Skin; and I think, fo far as I
have been able to obferve, thofe People have
been lefs fubject to relapfe into Fevers where
this Caution has been ufed, than where it has
been neglected.   That

That Species of the Itch where it forms small Ulcers or Pustules in the Skin, is the worst Kind, and most contagious, and seems to take its Rise from the common Itch continuing long, and making its Way deeper into the Skin. The Cure is the same, only this requires more frequent Unctions, and those to be continued longer, than before the Disorder has taken such deep Root.

It is no uncommon Thing to see the Itch appear again, some Weeks after it has seemingly been cured by the Use of sulphureous Unctions; which most commonly happened to those who were in too great a Hurry to get well, and left off the Use of the Unctions too soon. Such Returns of the Itch were generally cured by the Repetition of the same Treatment as before.

TABLE

TABLE of DIET.

The following is a Copy of the Table of Diet which was uſed in the Hoſpital all the Time I was with the Troops in *Germany*:

	Breakfaſt.	*Dinner.*	*Supper.*
Full Diet,	One Pint of Rice Gruel ; made with two Ounces of Rice, one Spoonful of fine Flower, a little common Salt, and fine Sugar.	One Pound of Meat.	As Breakfaſt.
Middle Diet,	As above.	One Pint of Broth, Half a Pound of Meat.	As above.
Low Diet,	As above, or according to the Patient's Stomach or Indiſpoſition.	One Pint of Broth; or Half a Pint of Panado, with two Spoonfuls of Wine, and a Quarter of an Ounce of fine Sugar.	As Breakfaſt.

T   The

The daily Allowance of Bread was a Pound to thofe on full and middle Diet, and Half a Pound to thofe on low Diet, or a Pound, if fo ordered by the Phyfician.

Thofe on full and middle Diet were allowed daily three Pints of Barley or Rice Water; to each Pint of which were added two Spoonfuls of Brandy, and a Quarter of an Ounce of Lump Sugar. Small Beer was mentioned in the Diet Table; but this we could never have good; and therefore was not ufed.

Thofe on low Diet were allowed Barley or Rice Water; to which fome Wine or Brandy was occafionally added, if ordered fo by the Phyfician.

Befides this, the Phyfician might order an additional Quantity of Wine, Brandy, or Milk, or Water Gruel, or any other Articles which he thought proper for the Sick under his Care, and which could be got eafily.

P H A R-

PHARMACOPOEIA

IN USUM

Nosocomii Regii Militaris Britanici.

M D C C L X I.

PHARMACOPOEIA

IN USUM

Nofocomii Regii Militaris.

Ann. MDCCLXI.

AQUÆ SIMPLICES ET SPIRITUOSÆ.

AQUA Alexeteria.
—— Bacc. Juniperi.
————— Cinnamomi.
————— Menthæ vulgaris.
————— Menthæ piperitidis.
————— Nucis mofchatæ.
————— Pulegii.
————— Rutæ.

Vel aliæ aquæ hujus generis præparari poffint, terendo in mortario vitreo elaeofacchara
præparata, cum oleis effentialibus, et facchari
albi 12ᵗᵃ quantitate; et dein addendo aquæ

Fontanæ

fontanæ vel fpiritus vini tenuis quantitatem fufficientem (*a*).

Aqua calcis fimp.   Ph. Lond.
Dofis a lib. i. ad lib. ij. in die.

Aqua Hordeata.   Ph. Lond.
Utenda pro potu.

B O L U S.

Bolus anodynus aftringens.
R Theriacæ andromachi, drachm. dimid.
opii, gr. i. M. pro dofi femel vel bis die.

Bolus e rheo cum mercurio.
R Pulv. rhei, gr. xxv. calomel, gr. v. fyrup
facchari, q. s.

Bolus e calomel.
R Calomel gr. v. conferv. rofar. fcrup i. M.

(*a*) Such *Elaeofacchara* (as they are called), made by rubbing the effential Oils with twelve Times the Quantity of Sugar, may at all Times be prepared at the fixed Hofpital, and carried about with the flying Hofpital, much more conveniently than the fimple or compound Waters themfelves.

Bolus

Bolus mercurialis.

℞ Argenti vivi, gr. x. extingue in balſam copaivi, q. s. et adde conſerv. roſar. q. s.

Bolus e ſcordio cum rheo.

℞ Elect. e ſcordio, ſcrup. i. pulv. Rhei, gr. x. ſyrup, q. s. ut fiat bolus ſumendus ſemel, bis, terve die.

COLLYRIA.

Collyrium ſaturninum.

℞ Sacchari ſaturni, ſalis ammoniaci crudi ana gr. vi. ſolve in aq. fontanæ, unc. xij. adde pro re nata tinct. thebaicæ, drachm. i.

Collyrium vitriolicum.

℞ Vitrioli albi, drachm. ſs. ſolve in aq. fon-tanæ, lib. i.

Confectio cardiaca. Ph. Lond.
Conſerva cynoſbat. Ph. Lond.
Conſerva roſar. Ph. Lond.

T 4 D E-

DECOCTA.

Decoctum album. Ph. Lond. utendum pro potu.

Decoctum arabicum.

℞ Gum. aribici, unc. dimid. coque in aq. hordeatæ bullientis, lib. ij. ad folutionem Gummi. utend. pro potu.—addi poffit pro re nata fpirit. nitri dulcis, drachm. ij.

Dococtum corticis Peruviani.

℞ Cort. Peruv. crafs. pulv. unc. i. coque in aq. fontan, lib. iij. ad lib. ij. Colaturæ adde tinct. cort. Peruv, unc. i. fpirit vini Gallici fefcunc. Dofis ab uncia i. ad unc. iv. bis ter. quaterve die.

Decoctum cort. cum ferpentaria.

Fit addendo decocto cort. Peruv. fub finem coctionis, rad. ferpentariæ virgin. contus. unc. dimid. Dofis ab unc. i. ad unc. iij. ter quaterve die.

Decoct. commun. pro clyfter.

℞ Flor. vel herb. chamamel. unc. i. coque in aq. fontan, lib. i.fs. ad lib. i, & cola.

De-

Decoctum ligni guaiaci.

℞ Ligni guaiaci ras. lib. ſs. aq. fontanæ bullientis, cong. ij. macera per noctem; mane coque ad congium. i. & cola; Capiat a lib. ſs. ad lib. ij. die.

Decoctum nitroſum.

℞ Coccinel. ſcrupul. i. coque in aq. fontan. lib. ijſs. ad lib. ij. & dein adde ſalis nitri, unc. i. ſacchar. albi ſeſcunc. Colaturæ addi poſſit pro re nata aq. alicujus ſpirit. unc. ij. Doſis ab unc. i. ad unc. iv. 4tis vel 6tis horis.

Decoctum pectorale.

℞ Fol. herb. malvæ, unc. ij. ſeminum lini, unc. dimid. coque in aq. fontan. lib. ivſs. ad lib. iv. addendo ſub finem coctionis rad glycyrrhiz ſeſcunc. vel mellis optimi, unc. i. Cola pro potu.—Adde pro re nata aceti, ſeſcunc.

Decoctum rad. ſarſaparillæ.

℞ Rad. ſarſaparillæ, unc. iij. coque in aq. fontan. lib. iij. ad lib. ij. adde ſub finem coctionis ligni ſaſafras, drachm. i. rad. glycyrrhizæ,
drachm.

drachm. ij.   Colaturæ capiat a lib. i. ad lib. ij. in die.—Adde pro re nata vini antimonialis, drachm. ij.

E L E C T A R I A.

Elect. aftringens balfamicum.

R Specier. e fcordio, pulv. e tragacanth comp. ana unc. i. tincturæ thebaicæ, drachm. ij. fyrup facchari, q. s. ut fiat elect. Dofis ad molem N. M. bis, ter. quaterve in die.

Elect. corticis Peruviani.

R Pulv. cort. Peruv. unc. iv. fyrup facchari, q. s. Dofis a fcrup. i. ad drachm. unam, bis, ter, 4r. 6ties. vel decies die.

Elect. corticis anodynum.

R Elect. cort. Peruv. unc. 1nam. elect. e fcordio unciam dimidiam, vel tinct. thebaicæ fcrup. ij.

Elect. corticis aftringens.

R Elect. cort. Peruv. femunc. pulv. rad. tormentil, lapidis cancror. ppt. fingulorum, drachm. i. fyrup, q. s.

Elect.

Elect. cort. cum serpentaria.

℞ Elect. cort. Peruv. unc. i. pulv. rad. serpentar. virgin. cort. canel. alb. ana, drachm ij. syrup. q. s.

Elect. cort. cum sale ammoniac.

℞ Elect. cort. Peruv. sescunciam. sal. ammon. crud. drachm. i.

Elect. e baccis lauri. Ph. Lond.
Elect. lenitiv. Ph. Lond.

Elect. lenitivum cum sulphure.

℞ Elect. lenitiv. lib. ss. flor. sulphuris, unc. ij. Dosis, moles, N. M. vel ad semunc. pro re nata.

Elect. lenitivum compositum.

℞ Elect. lenitiv. lib. i. pulv. jalap. unc. i. sal. nitri, drachm. ij. syrup. q. s. Dosis a drach. i. ad drach. iv. pro r. n.

Elect. lenitivum balsamicum.

℞ Elect. lenitiv. comp. unc. ij. balf. copaiv. unc. i. gum guaiac. unc. ss. M. Dosis, cochleare theæ, h. s. vel mane & vesperi.

Electuar.

Electuar. e fcordio vel diafcordium. Ph. Lond.

Elect. e fpermat. ceti.

℞ Balfam Peruv. unc. iᵐ. mifce optime cum mucilag. gum arab. fefcunciam & adde fpermat. ceti, conferv. rofar. ana unc. xij. fyrup facchar. q. s. dofis, a dimidiâ drachma bis die ad drachm. iᵐ. quater vel fexties die.

Elect. ftomachicum.

℞ Conferv. cynofbat. unc. iv. pulv. rad. zinziber. drachm. ij. canell. alb. unc. i. rubigin. martis, drachm. ij. fyrup. q. s. dofis a fcrup. i. bis terve die ad femidrach. 4ᵗⁱˢ horis.

Elect. e fcammon. Ph. Lond.

E L I X I R.

Elix aloes. Ph. Lond.

Elix. paregoricum. Ph. Lond.

Elix. vitrioli acid. Ph. Lond.

E N E-

E N E M A T A.

Enema commune laxativ.

℞ Aq. fontan. calid. unc. xij. elect. lenitiv.
femunc. fal. cathartici amari, unc. ſ. M.

Enema commun. oleos.

℞ Aq. fontan. bullient. unc. x. mucilag. gum
arabic. unc. iᵐ. olei olivar. unc. ij. adde pro re
nata elect. e ſcord. drachm. ij. vel. tinct. thebaic, drachm. i.

Enema ex amylo.

℞ Aq. fontan. calid. unc. iv. gelatin. amyli,
unc. v. elect. e ſcord. drachm. i. M.

Enema terebinth.

℞ Terebinth commun. drachm. vi. ſolve in
vitello ovi & adde enemat. oleos. unc. x.

Emplaſtrum veſicatorium. Ph. Lond.

F O T U S.

Fotus communis.

℞ Fol. malv. flor. chamamel. ſingulorum,
m. i. coque in aq. fontan. q. s.

Totus

Fotus commun. fpirit.

℞ Fotus commun. lib. ij. aceti, lib. i. fpirit.
vini tenuis, lib. ſs. M. pro fotu.

Fotus cum ſale ammoniac.

℞ Fotus commun. lib. ij. ſal ammoniac crud.
unc. i.

Fotus volatilis.

℞ Fotus commun. q. s. aſperge panno ſta-
tim ante applicationem ſpiritus ſal. ammoniac;
q. s.

GARGARISMATA.

Gargariſma commune.

℞ Aq. hordeat. unc. xij. ſal. nitri, drachm. i.
mellis ſemunc. M. adde pro re nata ſpirit. vin.
unciam i.

Gargariſma acidum.

℞ Aq. hordeat. unc. xij. ſpirit. vini gallici,
unc. i. aceti ſeſcunc. tinɕt. myrrhæ, drachm. ij.
M.

Gargariſma volatile.

℞ Aq. hordeat. unc. xij. ſpirit. vin gallic:
unc. ij. ſal. vol. ammoniaci, drachm. i. M.

GUT-

GUTTÆ ANTIMONIALES ANODYNÆ.

℞ Vini antimonialis, unc. i_m. tinct. thebaic. drachm. ij. dosis a gutt. 30 ad 40 bis terve die, vel a gutt. 60 ad 140, h. s. in potu tepido.

H A U S T U S.

Hauftus fimplex.
℞ Aq. fontan. fefcunc. fpirit. vini gallici drachm. i. fs. facchar alb. drachm. dimidiam M.—Hauftus præparari poffit aqua aliqua fimp. et fpirit. loco aq. fontan. & fpirit. vini gallici pro re nata.

Hauftus anodyhus.
℞ Hauft. fimp. fefcunc. tinct. thebaic. gutt. xx. M.

Hauftus camphoratus.
℞ Camphoræ, gr. iij. tere in mortario cum facchar. alb. drach. dimid. & dein adde mucilag. gum arabici, drachm. ij. hauft. fimp. fefcunciam. M. f. a. Dofis repetenda, 4ta. vel 6ta. quaque hora.

Hauft.

Hauſt. emetic. antimonialis.

℞ Vini antimonialis ſemunciam. Dari poſſit ad drachm. x. pro r. n.

Hauſt. emeticus ſcilliticus.

℞ Oxymel. ſcillit. drachm. x. aq. fontan. ſemunc. pulv. rad. ipecacoan. gr. vi.

Hauſtus cardiacus.

℞ Hauſt. ſimp. ſeſcunciam confeɕt. cardiac. ſcrup. im. M. f. hauſtus repetendus 4tis. vel 6tis. horis—adde pro re nata ſp. lavend. comp. dr. i.

Hauſtus cardiacus oleoſus.

℞ Ol. eſſential. menth. gutt. ij. tere in mortario vitreo cum ſacchar. alb. drachm. dimid. & adde hauſt. ſimplicis ſeſcunc. tinɕt. ſtomachic. drachm. i. M.—adde pro re nata tinɕtur. thebaic. gutt. x.

Hauſtus lixivioſus anodynus.

℞ Hauſt. ſimp. ſeſcunciam, lixivii tartari, drachmam dimidiam tinɕturæ thebaicæ, gutt. xx. cap. h. s. vel mane & veſperi.

Hauſtus

Hauftus e mithridatio.

R Hauft. fimp. fefcunc. mithridat. fcrup. i.
aceti vin. drachm. iij. dofis repetenda 4tis. vel.
6tis, horis.

Hauftus oleofus communis.

R Mucilagin. gum arabici, drachm. iv. ol.
olivar, drachm. v. mifce s. a. & adde hauft.
fimp. fefcunciam. Repet. 4 . vel 6tis. horis.

Hauftus oleofus cum rheo.

R Hauft. oleos. communis, unc. ij. tinct.
rhei fefcunc. vel pulv. rhei, gr. xxv. tinct. thebaic gutt. xv. M. fiat hauftus fumendus vel h. s.
vel primo mane.

Hauftus purgans.

R Infuf. fenæ, unc. iij. fal. glauber. drachm.
iij. fpirit. vin. gallici, drachm. ij. facchar. alb.
drachm. dimid. capiat mane.

Hauftus falinus communis.

R Aceti vinofi vel fucc. limonum femunciam,
fal. abfynth. fcrup. i. vel ad faturationem, hauft.
fimp. fefcunciam adde pro re nata pulv. contra-

U   yerv.

yerv. comp. ſcrup. i. vel pulv. contrayerv. cum nitro, ſcrup. ij.—Hauſtus præparari poſſit cum ſalis diuretici drachma dimid. loco acidi & ſalis abſynthii. Doſis repetend. 3^{tis}. 4^{tiis}. vel 6^{tis}. horis — Eodem modo fit hauſtus cum ſpirit. mindereri uncia dimidiâ.

Hauſt. ſalin. cum confect. cardiaca.

℞ Hauſt. ſalin. commun. unc. ij. confect. cardiac. ſcrup: i. M. repet. 4^{tis}. vel 6^{tis}. horis.

Hauſt. ſalin. cum mithridatio.

℞ Hauſt. ſalin. commun. unc. ij. mithridatii, ſcrup. i. M. ſumend. 4^{tis}. vel 6^{tis}. horis.

Hauſtus ſalin. cum rheo.

℞ Hauſt. ſalin. com. uncias ij. pulv. rhei, gr. xxv. M. capiat mane.

Hauſtus ſalin. cum phu.

℞ Hauſt. ſalin. commun. unc. ij. pulv. rad. valerian. ſylveſtris, ſcrup. ij. Doſis repetend. 2^{dis}. 4^{tis}. vel 6^{tis}. horis.

Hauſt. ſalinus ſuccinatus.

℞ Hauſt. ſalin. commun. unc. ij. ſal ſuccini, pulv.

pulv. caſtorei ſingulorum, gr. x. H. repetend.
4tis. vel 6tis. horis.

Hauſt. ſalinus purg. oleoſus.

R Mannæ opt. ſemunc. olei olivar. drachm.
vi. vitelli ovi q. s. tere in mortario, addendo
paulatim ſal cathartici amari, unc. i. ſolutam in
aq. fontan. calid. unc. iij. ſpirit. vini gallici vel
aq. alicujus ſpirituoſæ, drachm. iij. M. s. a pro
doſi matutino.

Hauſtus volatilis.

R Hauſt. ſimp. ſeſcunciam ſal. vol. c. cervi;
gr. x. M. H. repet. 4tis. vel 6tis. horis.

I N F U S A.

Infuſum amarum. Ph. Lond. Addi poſſit pro
re nata in præparando ſpirit. vini tenuis, lib. ſs.
ad lib. ij. infuſi. Doſis ab unc. ina. bis die ad
unc. ij. ter. die.

Infuſum raphani ruſticani.

R Rad. raphani ruſticani, unc. ij. baccar.
juniper, unc. inam. cort. canell. alb. drachm. ij.

aq.

aq. fontan. bullient, lib. iv. infunde per noctem
leni calore.   Colaturæ adde fpirit. vini gallici
unc. iv. Dofis ab. unc. i. bis terve die ad unc.
iv. 6tis. horis.

Infufum fenæ commun. Ph. Lond.

JULEPUM E MOSCHO.

℞ Mofch. drachmam im. tere optime in
mortario cum facchar. alb. drachm. iij. & adde
mucilagin. gum arab. dr. iv.   Hauft. fimp.
unc. vi. Dofis unc. ij. 4tis. vel 6tis. horis.

L I N C T U S.

℞ Conferv. cynofbat. unc. iv. ol. olivar. fyrup.
facchari vel mellis ana unc. ij. adde pro re nata
fpirit. vitrioli tenuis, drachm. iv.   Dofis cochleare theæ urgente tuffi.

L I N I M E N T A.

Liniment. faponaceum. Ph. Lond.

Lini-

Linimentum camphoratum.

R Olei olivar. unc. ij. camphoræ, drachm. ij. M.

Linimentum volatile. Ph. Lond.

Linimentum volatile commune.

R Olei olivar. unc. iij. fpiritus falis ammo-niaci, dr. vi. M.

M E L L A.

Mel cum borace.

R Mellis optimi, unc. i. pulv. fubtiliffim. boracis, dr. i. M.

Mel Ægyptiacum. Ph. Lond.

Mel rofaceum. Ph. Lond.

MITHRIDATUM. Ph. Lond.

M I X T U R Æ.

Mixtura acida communis.

R Hauft. fimp. unc. viij. fpirit. vitrioli te-nuis, fcrup. ij. vel ad gratam aciditatem. Dofis ab. unc. ij. ad unc. iv. 4^{tis}. vel 6^{tis}. horis.

Mixtura

Mixtura ammoniaca.

R Gum ammoniaci, drachm. i. folve in hauft. fimp. unc. vi. Dofis ab. unc. i. ad unc. ij. bis terve in die.

Mixtura ammon. cum oxymel.

R Mixt. ammoniac, unc. vi. oxymel fcillit. drachm. vi. Dofis a cochlear. i. ad unc. ii. ter. 4^{rve}. die.

Mixtura ammoniac. anodyna.

R Mixt. ammoniac. cum oxymel. unc. vi. tinct. thebaic. drachm. dimid. Dofis a cochlear. i. ad iv. 4^{tis}. vel 6^{tis}. horis.

Mixtura Campechenfis.

R Extract. ligni Campechenfis, drachm. iij. folve in hauft. fimplic. unc. vi. adde pro re nata tinct. thebaic. gutt. xxx. vel Philon. Londinen. drachm. i. Dofis ab. unc. i. ad unc. iij. bis, ter, 4^{rve}. die.

Mixtura fætida.

R G. afafætid. drachm. i. folve in hauft. fimp. unc. vi. Dofis ab. unc. i. ad unc. iij. 4^{r}. die.

Mixtura

Mixtura fætida volatilis.

℞ Mixt. fǽtid. unc. vi. fpirit. volat. fal.
ammon. drachm. i. Dofis ab. unc. i. ad unc.
ij. bis, ter, 4^{rve}. die.

Mixtura fracaftorii.

℞ Hauft. fimp. unc. viij. Eleft. e fcordio,
drachm. iv. Dofis ab. unc. i. ad unc. ij. 4^{tis}.
vel 6^{tis}. horis.

Mixtura japonica.

℞ Hauft. fimp. unc. vi. Tinft. japonic.
unc. i. adde pro re nata tinft. thebaic. dr. i.

Mixtura laxativa.

℞ Eleft. lenitiv. unc: i. Mannæ femunc.
coque in aq. fontan. unc. xvi. ad unc. xij. Colaturæ adde fal. cathartici amari. fefcunciam.
fpirit. vini gallici, unc. i. Dofis ab. unc. ij. ad
unc. xij.

Mixtura purg. antimonial.

℞ Eleft. lenitiv. fefcunc. mannæ femunc.
coque in aq. fontan. unc. xx. ad unc. xvi. &
dein folve tartar. emetici, gr. x. Colaturæ dofis ab. unc. i. ad unc. iv. omni hora vel omni

U 4 2da.

2da. vel 3^{tia}, vel 4ta. hora, donec laxetur alvus.

Mixtura oleofa volatilis.

R Hauft. fimp. unc. vi. ol. olivar. unc. iij. fpi-rit. volatil. falis ammoniaci drachmam 1^{nam}. M. Dofis ab. unc. i. ad unc. iij. 3^{tiis}. vel 4^{tis}. horis.

Mixtura fcillitica.

R Hauft. fimp. unc. vi. oxymel 'fcillitic. drachm. vi. Dofis a drachm. iv. ad unc. ij, bis, ter, 4^{rve}. die.

Mixtura e fpermat. ceti.

R Spermat. ceti, drachm. ij. folve in vitello ovi & adde hauft. fimp. unc. vi. adde,! pro re nata, tinct. thebaic. fcrup. ij. Dofis ab. unc. i. ad unc. ij. 4^{tis}. vel 6^{tis}, horis.

Mixtura e fpermat. ceti cum balfamo.

R Balfam. copaiv. drachm. ij. tere in mor-tario cum mucilag. gum arabici, drachm. iij. & dein adde mixtur. e fpermat. ceti, unc. vi. Do-fis ab. unc. i. ad unc. iij. 4^{tis}. vel 6^{tis}. horis,

M U-

MUCILAGO. G. ARABICI.

℞ G. arabici pulv. unc. iv. folve in aq. puræ
bullient. unc. x.

Oxymel fcillit. Ph. Lond.

Philonium Londinen. Ph. Lond.

P I L U L Æ.

Pilulæ fætidæ.
℞ Gum afafætid. myrrh. ana drachm. i. fapon.
alb. hifpan. drachm. ij. Tinct. fuliginis q. s.
Dofis a gr. x. ad drachm. dimid. bis terve die.

Pilulæ guaiac.
℞ Sapon. albi hifpanici femunc. gum. guaiac,
fcrup. iv. fyrup. q. s. Dofis a fcrup. i. ad
drachmam dimidiam bis terve die.

Pilulæ gummofæ. Ph. Lond.

Pilulæ mercuriales.
℞ Argenti vivi femunc. extingue in balfam.
copaiv. q. s. & adde pulv. glycyrrhiz. gum
guaiac.

guaiac. fingulorum, drachm. vi. fyrup. q. s. ut fiat maffa. Dofis a fcrup. fs. ad drachmam dimidiam femel vel bis die.

Pilulæ rufi. Ph. Lond.

Pilulæ faponaceæ. Ph. Lond.

Pilulæ faponaceæ cum rheo.

℞ Sapon. alb. hifpanici, drachm. vi. pulv. rhei, drachm. ij. fyrup. facchari q. s. Dofis a fcrup. i. ad fcrup. ij. bis terve die.

Pilulæ fcilliticæ.

℞ Pulv. glycyrhiz. rad. fcill. exficcat ana drachm. dimid. rad. zinziber. drachm. i. fapon. alb. hifpan. drachm. ij. fyrup. q. s. Dofis a gr. iv. ad. gr. xvi. bis terve die.

Pilulæ ftomachicæ.

℞ Pulv. canell. alb. drachm. ij. extract. rad. gentian. dr. i. mucilag. gum arabici q. s. Dofis a fcrup. i. ad drachmam dimid. bis die—adde pro re nata rubigin. martis drachmam dimid.

PUL-

P U L V E R E S.

Pulvis aftringens.

℞ Pulv. canell. alb. rad., tormentill. fingulorum, drachm. i. M. Dofis a fcrup. i. ad
drachm. i.

Pulvis aluminofus.

℞ Alumin. crud. terræ japonicæ ana partes
æquales dofis a gr. viij. ad drachmam dimidiam.

Pulv. anodynus Doveri.

℞ Sal. nitri, tartari vitriolati fingulorum, unc.
iv. in crucibulum candens injice, agitetur donec
deflagratio & fcintillatio definat, & adde opii
concifi, unc. i. & in pulverem redige addendo
rad. glycyrrhiz. ipecacoanhæ fubtiliffime pulver.
ana, unc. i. & dein probe mifceantur omnia.
Dofis a gr. x. ad fcrup. ij. vel ad drachmam
1^{nam}.

Pulvis antimonialis.

℞ Pulv. e chel. cancror. drachm. x. tartari
emetici, dr. i. M. fiat pulv. fubtiliffimus. Dofis a gr. iij. ad gr. x. 4ta. vel 6ta. quaque hora.

Pulvis

Pulvis cardiacus.

R Pulv. canell. alb. drachm. i. rad. zedoariæ, drachm. ij. rad. serpentar. drachm. i. M. dosis a scrup. i. ad drachm. i. 4tis. vel 6tis. horis.

Pulvis chamæmelinus.

R Pulv. flor. chamæmel. drachm iij. aluminis, g. myrrh. ana drachm. i. Dosis a scrup. i. ad scrup. ij.

Pulv. contrayerv. comp. Ph. Lond.

Pulv. contrayerv. cum nitro.

R Pulv. contrayerv. comp. unc. iv. salis nitri, drachm. i. M. Dosis a scrup. i. ad drachm. i. 4tis. vel 6tis. horis.

Pulvis emeticus.

R Pulv. ipecacoanhæ, scrup. i. tartar emetici, gr. ij. Dosis a gr. xi. ad gr. xxii.

Hiera picra. Ph. Lond.

Pulv. Ipecacuanhæ cum opio.

R Pulv. rad. ipecacoan. gr. x. opii, gr. ij. dosis a gr. iij. ad gr. xij.

Pulv.

Pulv. e jalapio.

℞ Pulv. rad. jalapii, drachm. vi: rad. zinzib. drachm. ij.   Dofis a fcrup. i. ad fcrup. ij.

Pulv. jalapii cum nitro.

℞ Pulv. rad. jalap. drachm. iv. falis nitri drachm. iᵐ.   Dofis a fcrup. i. ad fcrup. ij.

Magnefia alba.

Pulv. nitrofus.

℞ Pulv. e chel. cancror. drachm. iij. nitri, drachm. i. M.   Dofis a fcrup. i. ad fcrup. ij. vel ad drachmam. i.

Pulv. nitrofus camphoratus.

℞ Pulv. nitros, fcrup. ij. camphoræ, gr. v. M.   Dofis a fcrup. i. ad fcrup. ij.

Pulv. nitrofus cum gum guaiac.

℞ Sal. nitri, drachm. ij. gum guaiac. drachm. dimid.   Dofis a gr. v. ad drachm. dimid.

Pulv. plummeri.

℞ Calomel. fulph. aurat antimonii ana dr. ij.

tere

tere in mortario ut fiat pulv. fubtiliffimus.
Dofis a gr. ij. ad gr. x. vel ad fcrup. iᵐ.

Pulvis ftanni. Ph. Lond.

Pulv. e fpermat. ceti cum nitro.
℞ Spermat. ceti, drachm. ij. facchar. albi
fal. nitri ana unc. iᵐ. Dofis a fcrup. dimid. ad
drachmam i.

Pulv. e tragacanth. Ph. Lond.

SALES ACIDI.

PRÆPARATIONES.

Acida mineralia		PRÆPARATIONES	
Spir. vitrioli fortis			
——————tenuis	Spir. vitrioli dulcis		Æther.
Spiritus nitri	Spir. nitri dulcis		
Spir. falis marini	Spir. falis dulcis.		

Varietat. acid. vegit.
- Acetum.
- Spiritus aceti vel acetum diftillatum.
- Succus limonum.
- Chryftalli tartari.

Acid. anomal.
- Sal. fuccini.
- Sal. fedativus Hombergeri.

SALES

SALES ALCALINI.

Alcal. vegit. { Sal. abfynthii.
Sal. tartari.

Alcal. min. { Sal. alcali mineral. feu foda, feu natrum.

Alcal. vol. { Sal. volatilis c. cervi.
Sal. volatilis fal. ammoniaci.

SALES NEUTRI.

SALES NEUTRI, qui fiunt ex ALCALI   et   ACIDO.

Tartarus vitriol.	vegetab.	
Sal. glauberi	minerali	vitrioli.
Sal. am. vitrioli	volatili	
Sal. nit. com.	vegetab.	
Nit. cubicum	mineral.	nitri.
Sal.am.nitrofum	volatili.	
Sal.digeft. fylvii	vegetabil.	
— marin. com.	minerali	Sal. marini.
— ammon.com·	volatili	

Varietates falis neutri comp. ex alcal. & acid. vegitab. {

Sal. diureticus	vegetab.	aceti.	
Tartar. tartar.	veget. tartari	chryft. tartar.	Vegetabil. }
Sal.citratus com.	veget. abfynth·	fucc. limonum.	
Sal. de feignette	minerali	chryft. tartar.	
Spir. mindereri·	volatili	acet. diftillat.	

Hi

Hi omnes fales neutri præparari poffint pro ufu medico admifcendo Alcali & acidum ad faturationem ; alii vero in cryftallos redacti, s. a. commodius circumferuntur pro ufu militari ; alii ut *fal. citratus comm.* et *fpiritus mindereri* facilius præparantur ad mifcendo alcali & acidum ad faturationem pro re nata (*b*).

Solutio mercurii corrofivi fublimati.

℞ Mercur. corrofiv. fublimat. gr. vi. fpir. vini gallici, unc. xii. M. fiat folutio. Dofis a femunc ad unc. i. die.

Species aromaticæ. Ph. Lond.

———— e fcordio. Ph. Lond.

Tartar. emetic. Ph. Lond.

Theriaca andromachi. Ph. Lond.

(*b*) This Table of neutral Salts is nearly the fame as one I have feen, which was faid to be a Copy of that given yearly by Dr. *Cullen*, Profeffor of Chymiftry in the Univerfity of *Edinburgh*, to his Pupils ; and as that publifhed by Dr. *Vogel*, in his *Inftitutiones Chymiæ*, fect. 629. Thefe neutral Salts are likewife taken Notice of by *Macquer*, in his *Elemens de Chymie*, and other late chymical Authors.

TINC-

TINCTURÆ.

Tinctura amara. ⎤
———— corticis Puruv. ⎥
———— martis in ſp. ſal. ⎥
———— japonica. ⎥
———— melampodii. ⎥ ⎬ Pharm. Lond.
———— myrrhæ. ⎥
———— ſacra. ⎥
———— ſaturnina. ⎥
———— ſerpentariæ. ⎥
———— thebaica. ⎦

Tinctura rhei.

R Pulv. rad. rhei, unc. ij. ſemin. cardamom minor. decortic. ſemunc. vini alb. hiſp. lib. ij. ſp. vini gallici, unc. viij. digere ſine calore & cola. Doſis ab. unc. i. ad unc. iij.

Tinctura ſtomachica.

R Cort. canell. alb. ſemunc. cort. aurantior. unc. i. ſemin. cardam. minor. decort. drachm. ij. ſpirit. vini gallici lib. ij. digere ſine calore & cola. Doſis a ſemunc ad unc. i. bis terve die. —Adde pro re nata vin alb. hiſp. lib. i.

X   U N-

U N G U E N T A.

Unguenta cærulea vel mercurial. Ph. Lond.

Unguentum fulphuratum. Ph. Lond.

V I N A.

Vinum amarum.

―― antimoniale.   } Pharm. Lond.

―― chalybeatum.

VITRUM CERATUM ANTIMONII.

A N

A N

E S S A Y

ON THE

MEANS of Preserving the Health of SOLDIERS

on SERVICE.

AND

Conducting MILITARY HOSPITALS.

OF THE

Means of Preferving the Health of Soldiers on Service.

THE Life of *Britiſh* Soldiers on Service, in Time of War, is ſo very different from what they lead in Time of Peace, as to ſubjeƈt them to many Inconveniences and Diſeaſes.

In Time of Peace, Soldiers are quartered either in Towns or Garriſons, where they are under the Eye of their Officers, who take Care that they keep themſelves clean, and provided with Neceſſaries ; they lie either in private Houſes or in Barracks, where they have a good Bed, regular Meals of wholeſome Proviſions, and enjoy moſt of the other Neceſſaries of

X 3   Life

Life in common with the lower Clafs of People,
their Duty is eafy, they mount Guard but feldom, and in other Nights enjoy an undifturbed Reft.

Whereas, during the Time of an active Campaign, they are feldom in Houfes ; they lie in
Tents upon the Ground, which is often bare,
and at beft covered only with Straw and a
Blanket ; and fometimes they are obliged, after fatiguing Marches in wet Weather, to lie
on the bare Ground, without even a Tent to
cover them ; they muft ftand Centinel, and be
upon Pikets and other Out-Pofts in the Night,
during all Kinds of Weather ; befides performing long fatiguing Marches, and other military
Duties ; and when near an Enemy, they are
perhaps on Duty every fecond or third Night,
befides working Parties, and other Duties of
Fatigue ; and what Reft they have is interrupted by frequent Alarms.   They have often
but little Time or Convenience to make themfelves clean.   Provifions are fometimes fcarce,
and frequently on long Marches they have no
Opportunity of dreffing what they can get:
Water

Water is fometimes difficult to be come at, and
what is to be got, is bad. And it frequently
happens, that neither Beer, Wine, nor Spirits,
can be purchafed for Money. In fixed Camps,
they are often expofed to the putrid Effluvia
of dead Bodies, of dead Horfes, and other Animals, and of the Privies and Dung of the
Horfes (*a*); and, in fome Encampments, likewife to the unwholefome Vapours of marfhy
Ground, and of corrupt ftagnating Water: All
which, joined to the other Hardfhips and Inconveniences unavoidably attending a military
Life in Time of Service, often give Rife to numerous Difeafes, which weaken an Army in a
moft furprifing Manner; and therefore Commanders ought to ufe every Means in their

(*a*) In the Year 1760, the Men, who remained in the fixed
Camp about *Warbcurg*, were very unhealthy; while the Regiments who were detached to the *Lower Rhine*, under the
Command of the Hereditary Prince of *Brunfwick*, enjoyed a
much better State of Health; and notwithftanding their great
Fatigues, and the Lofs they fuftained at the Affair of *Kampen*,
were much ftronger when they rejoined the Army to go upon
the Winter Expedition into the Country of *Heffe*, than thofe
Regiments which had remained in the fixed Camp.

Power,

Power, confiftent with the neceffary military Operations, to preferve the Health of the Soldiers.

Difeafes are more or lefs frequent in Armies according as the Seafon is hot or cold, wet or dry; according to the Nature of the Climate, and the Time of the Year in which military Operations are carried on ; the Nature of the Ground on which the Army is encamped, or the Situation of the Towns or Villages in which they are cantonned ; the Cleannefs, Neatnefs, and Drynefs of the Camp, and of the Tents or Houfes in which the Soldiers are lodged ; according as the Men are fupplied with Provifions, and good Water, good Beer, Wine, or other fermented Liquors ; or are well cloathed, and well furnifhed with Straw and Blankets; in proportion as the Duty is more or lefs fevere; and to the Care taken of fuch as are attacked with Sicknefs.

Soldiers generally enjoy good Health in cold dry Weather, even during the Time of fevere Froft ; if they be kept in Exercife, be well cloathed, and well fupplied with Provifions and good

gcod Liquors, and with Wood; as the Troops,
both in *Germany* and *North America*, experienced during the late War : but Cold joined to
Moifture was obferved always to be productive
of Difeafes.

Nor is mere Heat of itfelf fuch an Enemy
to Health (*b*) as is generally apprehended; but
when joined to Moifture, is obferved to give
Rife to the moft fatal Diforders in the warm
Climates.

In our northern Climates the Winters are
cold, and the Weather variable; fometimes it
is cold and rainy, at other Times thick and
foggy; fometimes we have fair Weather and
Sunfhine, at other Times Froft and Snow;
and fometimes it happens that we have all thefe
different Sorts of Weather in the fame Day:
During this Seafon, Soldiers are fubject to
Coughs, Pleurifies, Peripneumonies, Rheumatifms, and other Diforders of the inflammatory

(*b*) This Dr. *Pringle* takes Notice of; and Mr. *Naefmith*
fays, he obferved it in Voyages to the *Eaft Indies*, which afford
the faireft Trials of this Kind. See Dr. *Lind's Effay on the
Means of Preferving the Health of Seamen*, 2d edit. note to
page 5.

Kind.

Kind. And in very intenfe Froft, they are
liable to have their Limbs benumbed with
Cold, and their Extremities Froft bit (as it is
called).

And where there is a Want of frefh Provifions, and they are obliged to live on falted
Meat, and cannot have Greens, Pot Herbs, Roots,
or other frefh Vegetables, nor be properly fupplied with Beer, Cyder, Wine, or other generous fermented Liquors, they, as well as Sailors,
are fubject to the Scurvy (c) ; efpecially if they
be encamped or quartered in low damp Places.

The beft Means of guarding againft inflammatory Diforders, and other Mifchiefs arifing
from Cold, whether in Camp or in Quarters,
is, to take Care that the Soldiers be well
cloathed ; that they lie dry, and be well provided with Straw and Blankets, and with
Wood ; and to prevent, as much as poffible,

(c) Dr. *Joh. Valint Willius,* Army Phyfician to the King of
Denmark, in his Treatife on Camp Difeafes, fays, you fcarce
find a Camp in thefe northern Countries in which the true
Scurvy, attended with ftinking Breath and eroded Gums, is
not to be obferved. *Cap.* iii. *fect.* iii.

their

their expofing themfelves to fudden changes from Heat to Cold.

In thefe northern Climates, it would be right to allow every Soldier on Service a Flannel Waiftcoat, a Pair of worfted Gloves, and a warm woollen Stock, or a Neckcloth, to wear when on Duty in cold and wet Weather, as foon as the Winter begins to fet in (*d*). Dr. *Pringle* mentions the Advantage the Troops received

---

(*d*) A Flannel Waiftcoat, worfted Gloves, and woollen Stock, or a Neckcloth, may be purchafed for about Half a Crown *per* Man, and would contribute to preferve the Lives of many; the recruiting of others, to fupply whofe Places, if they die, will coft the Government a great deal more than the Price of the Articles mentioned ; which for a Regiment of nine hundred Men, at the Rate of two Shillings and Six-Pence *per* Man, comes only to 112 *l.* 10 *s. per Ann.* Every Recruit fent from *England* to the Army in *Germany*, coft the Government at leaft twenty Guineas before he joined his Regiment ; and every fick Man fent to the general Hofpital, coft the Government at leaft fixteen Pence *per* Day, which is ten Pence above his Pay ; fo that, if we fuppofe the extraordinary Cleathing here mentioned would preferve only the Lives of nine Men to each Regiment yearly, and keep forty in Health who would otherwife be fick, we fee what great Gainers the Government will be in Point of Money at the Year's End ; befides preferving the Lives and Health of fo many Men.

from

from the Flannel Waiftcoats fupplied by the Quakers, in the Winter Campaign of 1745-6, in *Britain*; and thofe Regiments who had them for their Men towards the End of the Campaigns in *Germany*, found that they contributed greatly to keep the Men in Health. Officers ought to take particular Care that the Men be well provided with good ftrong Shoes and Stockings; and where the Troops remain late in the Field, if the Government allowed a Pair or two extraordinary of each to every Foot Soldier, it would be of great Ufe to the Service.

Blankets ought to be provided for each Tent, and thofe carried along with the Regiment, fo as to be always ready for the Men when they come to their Ground. During the late War in *Germany*, a Couple of Blankets were allowed for each Tent of the *Britifh* Troops, and each Company carried their Blankets covered with an Oil Cloth on a Horfe; fo that they were always up with the Regiments when they came to their Ground.

Each Regiment ought to be provided with a Number of Watch Coats fufficient to ferve the Centinels

Centinels who are to be on Camp Duty, or general Guards, in very cold and wet Weather. Some of the Regiments in *Germany* had fuch Coats, and found great Service from them.

In Winter Quarters, Soldiers are apt to make the Rooms in which they fit, and their Guard Rooms, as hot as poffible; efpecially in *Germany*, where the Inhabitants ufe clofe Stoves, inftead of open Fires; and continue in thefe warm Rooms till they are called out on Duty, when, by being expofed to fudden Cold, they are apt to be feized with Inflammations of the Breaft; and therefore Officers ought to examine carefully the Quarters and Guard Rooms allotted for their Men, and chufe them dry and comfortable, if poffible (*e*); but never to allow

(*e*) Dr. *Pringle* has very juftly obferved, that upper Stories are preferable to Ground Floors; and that all uninhabited large damp Houfes ought to be rejeﬅed. *Obfervat. on Difeafes of the Army*, part ii. chap. iii. feﬅ. 2.

If Neceffity obliges Officers to put up with fuch Places for their Men, Care ought to be taken to clean them well, and to air and dry them by Means of Fires, before the Soldiers go into them; and to fupply well the Men who are to lodge in them with Straw and Blankets, and with Wood or Turf.

the

the Men to keep them as hot as Ovens, by
Means of clofe Stoves, or other fuch Contrivances ; but to depend more on good warm
Cloathing, and dry Quarters, for guarding a-
gainft Difeafes, than upon artificial Heat. Many
of the Regiments in *Germany* made the People
in whofe Houfes their Men were quartered,
take down their Stoves, and ufe only open
Fires ; when there was no Danger of the Soldiers making their Quarters too warm, as
Wood was difficult to be got.

But although clofe Stoves are prejudicial in
fmall Rooms, yet when a Town is much
crowded, and Men are obliged to be lodged, in
Winter, in large Barns or Churches, or other
large open Places, the *German* Stoves may be
ufed with great Advantage in airing and drying fuch Places, and keeping them of a moderate Heat; efpecially if there be a Place in
them for an open Fire, or if they be of that
Kind which the *Germans* call *wynd Stoves,*
which have a Door opening into the Chamber
where the People are lodged ; or if there be
broken Windows, or any other Opening by
which

which a free Circulation of Air can be kept up
in the Men's Apartments.

In Winter, when the Weather is very cold
or wet, a Glafs of Brandy, or of the fpirituous
Tincture of the Bark, given to the Men as they
went upon Duty, efpecially in the Night, has
been found to be of great Ufe(*f*). Dr. *Pringle*
has very juftly obferved, that the Times of ftanding Centinel, and being upon Out-pofts, ought, if
poffible, to be fhortened at fuch Seafons; and
that Fires in the Rear of the Camp, for Men
coming off Duty to warm and dry themfelves
at, were found to be of great Service.

(*f*) Dr. *Pringle* has taken Notice, that it would be a right
Meafure to make an Allowance of Spirits to the Infantry on
Service; which certainly would be of great Ufe, and fave
many Mens Lives; and might be done at a fmall Expence to
the Government, if properly managed; as it would only be
requifite to make fuch an Allowance when the Troops are in
the Field, and to fuch Men as mount Guard in cold wet Weather, or at Nights in Garrifon Towns, during the Winter. If
ever fuch an Allowance be made, what Spirits are given to the
Men ought to be mixed with five or fix Times the Quantity of
Water; except when Men are to ftand Centinels, or to be upon
Out-Pofts, in a frofty Seafon, or in cold wet Weather; at which
Time a fmall Glafs of pure Spirits may be given them in Pre-
fence of the Officer or Serjeant of the Guard.

In

In Spring, and the latter End of Autumn, the Days are fometimes extremely hot, and the Nights cold and damp, and the Men expofed to thefe fudden Changes; at fuch Times, the Men who go upon Duty in the Night, ought to put on their Flannel Waiftcoats, and be warmer cloathed than in the Day; and ufe many of the Precautions practifed in Winter for the Prefervation of their Health.

In *North America*, when the Men were in the Field in very hard frofty Weather, Fires were lighted at the Ends of the Tents, and Centinels fet over them to prevent their doing Mifchief; and both in *Germany* and *North America*, when the Troops were in the Field without Tents, they cut down Wood and made large Fires, and the Soldiers lay down and flept round thefe Fires, with their Feet next to them; and Fires were lighted at all Out-pofts, where it could be done with Safety.

In *Germany*, when the Weather fet in rainy or cold towards the End of the Campaigns, and the Army was in a fixed Pofition, his Serene Highnefs Prince *Ferdinand* conftantly ordered

the

the Army to Hutt; which was done either by thatching their Tents, or building Hurdles, or digging Pitts, and covering and thatching them over. The Officers either built Hutts with Fire Places, or had Chimnies built to their Tents.

If, notwithſtanding all Precautions, Men upon Out-poſts ſhould be benumbed with Cold, or Froſt bit, as ſoon as they are brought into Camp or Quarters, their Extremities ought to be rubbed with Snow, or put into cold Water (*g*); and afterwards well dried, and wrapt up in Blankets; and warm mild Liquors given

(*g*) *Hildanus* relates a very remarkable Inſtance of the good Effeɛts of this Treatment. A Man was found quite ſtiff and frozen all over. He was put into cold Water, and immediately the icy Spicula were diſcharged from all Parts of his Body, ſo that he ſeemed covered with an icy Cruſt. He was then put into a warm Bed, and took a Cordial Draught, and a plentiful Sweat followed; after which he recovered with the Loſs of the laſt Joints of his Fingers and Toes. *De Gangræna*, cap. xiii. People who are benumbed with Cold in froſty Weather ought never to be brought immediately near a Fire; for that has been found either to cauſe immediate Death or Gangrenes of the Extremities; and even Apples and other Fruits which have been frozen, if brought immediately near a Fire, turn ſoft and rot; but if put into cold Water, throw out the icy Spicula, and re-cover, ſo as to be almoſt as good as before they were frozen.

Y   them

them to drink, and afterwards Cordials ; and, after fome Time, they may be brought near the Fire, or put to Bed. Dr. *Lind* (*b*) mentions one Caution to be ufed when Men are found in this Condition ; which is, not to give them immediately ftrong fpirituous Liquors, for that thofe often prove inftantaneoufly fatal; but to put them to Bed, and give warm Water Gruel, or fome other mild diluting Liquor, to drink ; after which, he fays, a Glafs of Spirits will prove lefs dangerous and more beneficial.

When Men are quartered or cantonned in Towns or Villages, whofe Situation is low and damp, and where frefh Meat and Vegetables are fcarce in Winter, and the Scurvy frequent among the lower Clafs of People ; Commanding Officers, at the Approach of Winter, ought to ufe their Endeavours to provide a Store of Potatoes, Onions, Cabbages, four Crout ; of pickled Cabbages, and other pickled Vegetables ; of Apples and other Fruits, preferved in different Forms, to be laid up, and fold out to

(*b*) *Means of Preferving the Health of Seamen,* 2d edition, page 19.

the

the Men at a cheap Rate during the Winter. They fhould contract, if poffible, with Butchers to furnifh the Men with frefh Meat (*i*), and endeavour to procure good fmall Beer, or Cyder or Wine in the Wine or Cyder Countries; or Spirits to be mixed with Water, and a fmall Proportion of Cream of Tartar or Vinegar; or fome other wholefome fermented Liquor for their Drink (*k*); and to put their Men into as dry comfortable Quarters as poffible.

In Times of War, when Men are fent upon Expeditions into warm Climates, great Care ought to be taken to embark fuch only as are in good Health; particular Regard ought to be paid to thofe who are picked up in the Streets, or have been taken out of the *Savoy*, or other

(*i*) The Regiments in *Germany* who kept their Butchers in Winter, and made Stoppages of the Mens Pay, and obliged them to take a certain Quantity of Meat daily, were much more healthy than thofe who ufed no Precaution of this Kind.

(*k*) In Places where the Articles here mentioned are at too high a Price for a Soldier's Pay, a fmall Allowance, from the Government, of fuch Things would contribute much to the Prefervation of the Mens Health in unwholefome Garrifons.

Y 2

Jails.

Jails. All dirty Rags from off fuch People
ought to be thrown away or burnt; and the
Men, after being well wafhed, and new cloathed, ought to be kept for a Fortnight or three
Weeks in fome Garrifon Town, or with their
Regiments, in open airy Places, that it may be
afcertained that they have no infectious Diforder
before they be put aboard the Tranfports.

All Ships allotted for Tranfports ought to
be well aired and purified, and every Thing
fitted up properly, before the Men are em-
barked. They ought to be provided with
Ventilators, or Wind Sails, to make a free Circulation of Air through the Veffel (*l*); and
they ought never to be crowded; but full
Room allowed for each Man, in Proportion to
the Length of the Voyage (*m*).

In

(*l*) See Dr. *Lind's Treatife on the Means of Preferving the
Health of Seamen in the Royal Navy*, where he takes Notice of
moft of the Articles here mentioned with regard to Tranfport
Ships in treating of Ships of War.

(*m*) When Ships are too much crowded with Men, if they
meet with a tedious Paffage, and hot moift clofe Weather, they
are often attacked with Difeafes which prove very fatal. Dr.
Lind,

In military Expeditions, Soldiers are put upon Ships Allowance; which, Dr. *Lind* very juſtly obſerves, ought not, in Voyages to the warm Climates, be made up ſo much of ſalted Beef and ſalted Pork (which always tend to the Putreſcent), as is the common Practice of the Navy; but that a greater Share of Biſcuit, Flour, Oatmeal, Goarts, Rice, and other Stores of that Kind, ought to be laid in; and a greater Proportion of them, and a Leſs of the ſalted Meat, diſtributed among the Men: And he is certainly in the Right, when he ſays, that a full Animal Diet, and tenacious Malt Liquors, are well adapted to the Conſtitution of our own, and of other northern Climates; and that Sailors who viſit' the *Greenland* Seas, and are

---

Lind, talking of Ships of War, ſays it is a Miſtake deſtructive to the Men to crowd too many of them together in a ſouthern Voyage, or in a hot Climate; as the Ship will be found, before the End of the Voyage, in more Diſtreſs for Want of Men, than ſhe would have been, had ſhe at firſt carried out only her proper Compliment. An additional Number is made, in order to ſupply an expected Mortality; but they generally increaſe that Mortality to double or triple their own Number. *Ibid. note to p.* 48.

Y 3 remarkable

remarkable for a voracious Appetite, and a
ftrong Digeftion of haid falted Meat, and the
coarfeft Fare, when fent to the *Weft Indies,*
foon become fenfible of a Decay of Appetite,
and find a full grofs falted Diet pernicious to
Health. " Inftinct (he fays) has taught the
" Natives between the Tropics to live chiefly
" on a Vegetable Diet, of Grains, Roots,
" and fubacid Fruits, with Plenty of diluting
" Liquors (*n*)."

A

(*n*) The following is the Diet eftablifhed for the Seamen of
his Majefty's Navy.

Every Man is allowed a Pound of Bifcuit, *Averdupoiz*
Weight, and a Gallon of Beer, *Wine Meafure, per* Day.

On *Sunday* and *Thurfday,* one Pound of Pork, and Half a
Pint of Peas, *Winchefter Meafure.*

On *Monday, Wednefday,* and *Friday,* one Pint of Oatmeal,
two Ounces of Butter, and four Ounces of Cheefe.

On *Tuefday* and *Saturday* two Pounds of Beef.

It is left to the Commanders of Squadrons to fhorten the
aforefaid Allowance of Provifions according to the Exigence
of the Service, taking Care that the Men be punctually paid
for the fame. As it is thought for the Benefit of the Service
to alter fome of the foregoing Particulars of Provifions in Ships
employed on foreign Voyages, it is to be obferved, that

A Pint of Wine, or Half a Pint of Rum, Arrack, or Brandy,
hold Proportion to a Gallon of Beer.

Four

A Store of Vegetables, fuch as Muftard Seed, Garlick, Onions, Potatoes, pickled Cabbages and other pickled Vegetables, four Crout and other Things of that Kind, which can be purchafed at a cheap Rate, and preferved for fome Months, ought to be laid in; which may be mixed with the Soops prepared for the Men, or given them to eat along with their falted Provifions.

A Quantity of Beer, Cyder, or Wine, ought to be put aboard, and a certain Allowance diftributed to each Man daily. When, for Want of thefe, Men are reduced to an Allowance of Spirits, they ought to be mixed with feven or eight Times the Quantity of Water, or

Four Pounds of Flour, or three Pounds of the fame with a Pound of Raifins, Half a Pound of Currans, or Half a Pound of Beef Suet pickled, are equal to a four Pound Piece of Beef, or two Pound Piece of Pork with Peas.

Half a Pound of Rice is equal to a Pint of Oatmeal.

A Pint of Olive Oil is equal to a Pound of Butter, or two Pounds of *Chefhire* Cheefe.

And Two-thirds of a Pound of *Chefhire* Cheefe is equal to a Pound of *Suffolk*.

If Soldiers are fent as Paffengers on board of King's Ships, or on board of Tranfports, their Allowance is generally but Two-thirds of the above.

Y 4   made

made into Punch, by the Mixture of Water and Moloffes, and the Juice of Lemons, before they are given to the Men; and, if Lemons cannot be got, Cream of Tartar, or Vinegar, ought to supply their Place; and it ought to be a Duty of one of the military Officers on board to fee the Punch made, and diftributed among the Men daily.

It would be right, on all Expeditions into warm Climates, to fend fome Sloops of War, or other armed Veffels, before the grand Fleet, to take up a Quantity of Wine that will keep, either at the *Madeira*, or other Wine Countries; and afterwards to go to any of our Settlements that are neareft the Place of Deftination, and to take in a Quantity of Limes, Lemons, Oranges, and other Fruits, and Vegetables which will keep for fome little Time; and of Spirits, live Stock, and other Provifions proper for the Army; and then to meet the Fleet at the general Rendezvous. When once a Landing is made good, thefe Veffels, after having unloaded their Cargoes, may either be employed on other Services, or kept conftantly going and coming for whatever Stores or Provifions are wanted for the Army or Fleet.

A fufficient

A fufficient Quantity of Vinegar ought to be put on board of each Tranfport, both for the Men to eat with their Victuals, and likewife for fumigating and wafhing between Decks occafionally. And a Quantity of Moloffes, or coarfe brown Sugar, and of Lemons, or their infpiffated Juice, or Cream of Tartar, ought to be allowed for making the Punch, as well as for other Purpofes.

If the Water become fœtid, the Quantity to be ufed in the Day ought to be fweetened by Means of the Ventilator contrived by the ingenious Dr. *Hales* (*o*) for that Purpofe.

The Men ought to be brought upon Deck, and Roll called two or three Times a Day; they fhould be made to comb their Hair, and wafh their Hands and Face every Day, and to

(*o*) This Ventilator is no more than a long Tube, with a Tin Box, about fix Inches wide and four high, with a Number of Holes at the Top, fixed at one End; and this Box is put down to the Bottom of the Water, and the Nofe of a Pair of Bellows fixed to the other End of the Tube, which is above the Water; by working the Bellows, frefh Air is driven through the whole Body of Water, the putrid Effluvia are evaporated and difperfed, and the Water becomes fweet in a very fhort Time.

fhift

shift themselves sometimes, if poffible ; and in every respect keep themselves as clean as the Nature of the Service will admit ; and proper Exercises should be contrived, to keep them in Health.

All the Parts of the Ship ought to be kept very neat and clean ; and the Hold, and all between Decks, ought to be scraped and swept daily ; and every Morning, in fair Weather, ought likewise to be washed, and afterwards sprinkled or washed with warm Vinegar, while the Men are upon Deck (*p*).

When the Weather will permit, Fires of dried Wood may be lighted in Iron Kettles between Decks, and Centinels set over them, and the Fires sprinkled with Rosin or Bits of Rope dipt in Tar, or with some cheap Aromatic ; and these Fires may be carried into all the Parts of the Ship that Safety will permit, in order to dry and purify the Air (*q*). After this

(*p*) This ought always to be done in the Morning, that all the Parts of the Ship may have Time to dry before the Men go to rest in their Births at Night ; but it ought never to be done after Sun-set.

(*q*) It has been propofed, that the Air in Ships of War should be

this Operation all the Ports and Hatchways thould be opened, and the Air in all the Parts of the Ship often renewed by working the Ventilators.

The Mens Hammocks and Beds ought to be brought up upon Deck in fair Weather, and well aired, and afterwards put in their Places, and Fires lighted below Decks.

When Troops, sent on an Expedition into warm Climates, arrive at the Place of their Destination, particular Care should be taken to guard them against the Diseases peculiar to such Climates, which are different from those common to our more northern Latitudes.

Dr. *Lind* says, that People coming first from a cold into a hot Climate are apt to have plethoric Symptoms ; a Pain of the Head, Giddiness, a Sense of Weight, and Fulness of the Breast, and a slight Inflammation of the *tunica conjunctiva* ; and that some are apt to be seized with ardent Fevers and Diarrhœas. And all Practitioners have observed, that New-Comers

be purified in this Way both by Dr. *Lind* and by Monf. *de Hamel de Monceau.*

into

into warm Climates are at firſt liable to Fevers
tending to the Ardent, and are very ſubjeƈt to
Fevers of the remitting and intermitting Kind,
which are the Endemics of all warm Countries at certain Seaſons of the Year; and after
ſome Time they are apt to fall into Fluxes,
the Yellow Fever, and other Diſeaſes depending on a putreſcent State of the Juices. In military Expeditions theſe Diſorders are liable to
be complicated with Fevers of the Malignant
or Hoſpital Kind, if Care is not taken to prevent it. And nothing has been found to be
more produƈtive of Diſeaſes in thoſe warm Climates, than indulging freely in the Uſe of Spirits
and other ſtrong fermented Liquors; expoſing
one's ſelf to the Damps, eſpecially lying on the
Ground after the Dews fall; and working hard,
or uſing violent Exerciſe in the Heat of the
Day.

The beſt Preſervatives againſt Diſeaſes in
warm Climates have been found to be,—
1. Temperance; a Diet of light and eaſy Di-
geſtion, compoſed more of vegetable than of
animal Food; ſuch as a ſmall Portion of freſh
Meat,

Meat, joined with a fufficient Quantity of Vegetables; Rice, *Indian* Corn, and other Grains,
and Roots of various Kinds, prepared in different Forms; well baked Bread; the moderate
Ufe of ripe Fruits; and the free Ufe of mild
cooling fubacid Liquors, joined with a fmall
Proportion of vinous or fpirituous Liquors;
carefully avoiding the too liberal Ufe of Wine,
Spirits, or other ftrong fermented Liquors.—
2. Great Care not to expofe one's felf to the
Damps of the Night, nor lie down to fleep on
the Grafs, or in woody moift Places, in the
Day; and to avoid all violent Exercife in the
Heat of the Sun.—3. Such Means as tend to
fupport the Spirits; for Chearfulnefs has been
obferved to contribute as much to the Prefervation of Health, as Fear and Dejection of Spirits to the Production of Difeafes.—4. Keeping
the Body clean, and bathing frequently in the
Sea, or in a River, in the Morning.

And therefore, in warm Climates, Officers
ought to be particularly careful to keep their
Men fober and temperate; to procure them
good Bread, and Plenty of Vegetables and frefh
Meat,

Meat, if possible; and where no other but salted Meat can be got, to make them boil a small Proportion of it in their Camp Kettles, along with Onions, Goarts, Rice, Carrots, Turnips, Greens, or any other wholesome Roots or Herbs which the Country affords, of they can get, and of these to prepare a good wholesome Soop for themselves; and where there is Plenty of the ripe acescent Fruits, which are reckoned wholesome, to distribute a moderate Quantity among the Soldiers daily, which will both help to preserve their Health, and prevent them from privately stealing and eating large Quantities to the Prejudice of their Health.—To encourage their Men, and keep up their Spirits.

They should also prevent, as much as possible, the too free Use of Wine, Spirits, or other strong fermented Liquors; and in Wine Countries give every Man a daily Allowance of Wine, to be mixed with Water for his common Drink; and in Countries where nothing but Spirits can be got, make the Spirit be mixed with Water, or made into a very weak Punch, before it is given to the Men, as Lemons, Oranges,

Limes,

Limes, and other Fruits proper for this Purpofe, are generally to be had in moſt warm Countries.

They ſhould be careful not to march their Men in the Heat of the Day, nor order them upon Duty where they muſt ſtand expoſed to the Dews and Damps of the Night, unlefs where the military Operations abſolutely re- quire it.

They ſhould endeavour to make the Bottom of the Tents be covered with Straw, or dried Leaves of Trees, or dried Reeds, and with Blan- kets (r), for the Men to lie upon.

The Time of ſtanding Centinel, and being upon Out-poſts, if poſſible, ſhould be ſhort, where Men are expoſed to the ſcorching Heat of the Sun ; and when Men are upon Out-poſts in the Night, it ſhould be recommended to them to lie down on the Ground as little as poſſible ; and if they do it, to chuſe a dry

(r) A ſufficient Store of Blankets has often been neglefted to be carried out in Expeditions into warm Climates; but Blankets are no-where more neceſſary, as it is very prejudicial to the Health of Soldiers to be obliged to lie down on the bare Ground ; and Straw, dried Reeds, and other ſuch Things, are often difficult to be got in the warm Climates.

Place ;

Place ; and, where it can be done, to have it covered with Straw or a Blanket, and to have fome light Covering to defend them from the Dews.

The Tents fhould be covered with Boughs of Trees, and the Men fhould be ordered fometimes to ftrike them in the Middle of the Day; and air well every Thing within them.

The Men fhould be obliged to keep themfelves neat and clean; to comb their Hair, and change their Linen often ; and if the Camp be near the Sea, or a large River, they ought to bathe themfelves as often as the Nature of the Service will permit. However the following Caution, mentioned by Dr. *Lind*, ought to be obferved, which is, not to go into the cold Bath when overheated with Work or Liquor, or when the Stomach is full, or when a critical Eruption, called the prickly Heat, appears on the Skin (*s*).

When

(*s*) Dr. *Lind* fays, the Ufe of the cold Bath, either in Tubs under the Forecaftle, or to dip in the Sea early in the Morning, has been found extremely beneficial in warm Weather and hot Countries ; and that he can affirm, from his own Experience in
hot

When Men are feized with inflammatory Symptoms on entering into warm Climates, they may be blooded freely : Afterwards they do not eafily bear fuch copious Evacuations, but rather require to have them made in fmaller Quantities, and very early and frequent, as Inflammations make a rapid Progrefs in warm Countries. Dr. *Lind* fays, many Practitioners difapprove of Blood letting in the Countries lying under the Torrid Zone, on a Suppofition that the Blood is too much diffolved; but he thinks that this Rule will admit of many Exceptions ; and that Sailors *(and confequently Soldiers)*, being ftrong and robuft, and expofed to greater Viciffitudes of Heat and Cold, and more Exceffes, and other Accidents in general, bear freer Bleeding than any other Set of People.

hot Climates, that many Diarrhœas and other Complaints, the pure and fole Effect of an unufual and great Heat (relaxing the Syftem of the Solids, and occafioning a Colliquation of the Animal Juices), have not only been cured by cold Bathing ; but their Return, and even the Attack of fuch Difeafes, effectually prevented by it. *Ibid.* p. 44, &c.

Z   After

After fome Time, the Difeafes in thefe warm Climates tend to the putrid Kind, and muft be treated as fuch.

In all Countries, and in all **Climates**, great Care ought to be taken in chufing the Ground on which Men are to encamp. Dry high Grounds, expofed to the Winds, where there is a free Current of Air, and which lie at a Diftance from Marfhes, ftagnating Water, and large Woods, are generally healthful in very different Climates (*t*). But Places fitu-ated low, where, on digging two or three Feet below the Surface of the Earth, you come to Water (*u*), and marfhy Grounds, and Places furrounded with corrupt ftagnating Water, are almoft always the contrary, and very unhealth-

(*t*) Mr. *du Hamel* fays, that the Air of the Ifland of *St. Do-mingo* is very fatal to *Europeans* ; but it is obferved that thofe People who inhabit the rifing Grounds are much lefs expofed to Difeafes than thofe who live in the Vallies. *Sur la fanté des Equipages*, art. i. p. 16.

(*u*) Ground may feem very dry and healthful, and yet be quite the contrary, as Dr. *Pringle* remarks is the Cafe in the Neighbourhood of *Bois le Duc*, in *Flanders*, where Water is found every-where at the Depth of two or three Feet from the Surface.

ful ;

ful ; as are often thofe Grounds which are fubject to be overflowed by large Rivers, and low
Places covered with Wood, where there is no
free Circulation of Air. However, it ought
to be obferved, that it is not the Neighbourhood of Water alone which is prejudicial, but
the watery Vapours which keep the Air perpetually moift, and the Exhalations of corrupt Effluvia, which render fuch Places unwholefome ;
for the Neighbourhood of Rivers, and of the
Sea, where the Tide ebbs and flows freely,
has no fuch Effect, where the Situation is dry
and airy; and thofe very unhealthy marfhy
Grounds often continue healthy in cold Weather, when their Waters are refrefhed with
Rains (*w*), and little or no moift putrid Exhalations rife from them ; though, as Dr. *Pringle*
obferves, in Summer and Autumn, when their
Waters begin to corrupt, and the Exhalation is
ftrong, they are always expofed to Difeafes ;

(*w*) Mr. *du Hamel* remarks, that Places which were formerly
very fubject to Difeafes have become healthful when the Water
which furrounded them was refrefhed by opening a Communication with the Sea. *Ibid.* art. i. p. 18.

and

and it is for this Reafon that fuch Places are always very unhealthy in warm Climates.

Hence, wheré the military Operations will permit, Commanders, if poffible, ought to chufe a dry Ground, whofe Situation is high, and which admits a free Current of Air, fuch as on the Banks of Rivers, where there is generally a Stream of frefh Air, and Plenty of frefh Water to fupply the Camp (*x*) ; taking Care to avoid the Neighbourhood of low márfhy Grounds, and corrupt ftagnating Waters, efpecially in Summer, and in hot Climates.

When Neceffity obliges Commanders to take Poft, or encamp in a wet or marfhy Ground, they fhould endeavour to make it as dry as poffible, by ordering Trenches to be cut for

(*x*) Dr. *Pringle* obferves, that where Grounds are equally dry, that the Camps are always moft healthful on the Banks of large Rivers ; becaufe in the hot Seafon Situations of this Kind have a Stream of frefh Air from the Water, tending to carry off both the moift and putrid Exhalations.—And in Cantonments we are not only to feek Villages removed from marfhy Grounds, but fuch as are leaft choaked with Plantations, and ftand higheft above fubterraneous Water. See his *Obfervat. on Difeafes of the Army*, 3d edit. p. 99.

Drains

Drains acrofs the Field and round the Mens
Tents; to fee that the Ground within the
Tents be well covered with Straw; to order
the Tents to be ftruck at Mid-Day, in dry
warm Weather, and the Men to dry and
air the Straw, and change it frequently; to
have a proper Supply of Blankets for the Men,
and to take Care that they be well cloathed,
efpecially thofe who go upon Duty in the
Nights; and, in the northern Climates, to have
Fires in proper Places for warming the Men
and drying their Cloaths, and for correcting the
Dampnefs of the Air (*y*).

In Countries lying under the Torrid Zone,
the Parts near the Sea Shore are often marfhy,

(*y*) The Negroes on the Coaft of *Guinea*, and fome of the
Indians, both of whom fleep on the Ground, have conftantly a
Fire producing a little Smoak burning in the Hutts where they
fleep, which corrects the Moifture of the Night, and renders
the Damp of the Earth lefs noxious; and during the Time of
the very unwholefome Fogs on the Coaft of *Guinea*, called Har-
mattans, which lay wafte whole Negroe Towns, the Smoak of
Wood, of pitched Staves, and fuch Things, are found to be
the beft Correctors of this thick Air. See Dr. *Lind's Means of
preferving the Health of Seamen.*

Z 3   or

or clofe and covered with Wood, or have fwampy Beaches, and are very unwholefome; and therefore where Soldiers aboard of Tranf-ports keep their Health, Commanders ought to be very careful not to allow them to land, till they come to the Place of their Deftination. Dr. *Lind* obferves, that Men commonly live more healthy in warm Climates at Sea, where the Air is dry and ferene, and the Heat mode-rated by refrefhing Breezes, than when they arrive in Harbours, or get within Reach of the noxious Vapours which arife from many Parts of the Land (*z*).

When Neceffity requires Parties to be landed for Wood or Water, or on other Duties, they fhould always be obliged to return and lie aboard at Night; and if that cannot be done, they fhould be cautioned to avoid lying down to fleep on the Grafs, where the Air is frefh, or they are expofed to the Dews; and to pitch their Tents on a rifing

(*z*) Dr. *Lind* fays, that it is conftantly obferved in unhealthy Harbours, that the Boats Crews employed in wooding and wa-tering the Ships, who are obliged to lie on Shore, fuffer moft. *Ibid.* p. 72.

Ground,

Ground, covered with Straw or dried Reeds, and a Blanket; and to ufe the other Precautions neceffary for encamping in thefe warm Climates; for where this Care has been neglected, the Confequences have frequently proved fatal (*a*). On unhealthful Coafts, the noxious Land Vapours often affect the Crews of Ships that run up into Rivers or Harbours, and caufe great Sicknefs; and therefore in fuch Places Ships fhould anchor at as great a Diftance from the Shore as can well be done, that they may be expofed to the Sea Breezes, and as much to

---

(*a*) A very remarkable Inftance of this we have related by Dr. *Lind.* In the Year 1739, in *Mahon* Harbour, a Party of Men were fent with the Coopers from Admiral *Haddock's* Fleet to refit and fill the Water Cafks, who, finding an artificial Cave dug out of a foft fandy Stone, put their bedding into it; every one who flept in this damp Place was infected with the Tertian Fever, then epidemic in *Minorca*, and not one in eight recovered. At the fame Time the Men aboard the Ships continued healthy; and others, who were afterwards fent on the fame Duty, enjoyed perfect Health by being obliged to fleep in their refpective Ships. He fays, he has known a whole Boat's Crew feized next Morning with bad Fevers by fleeping near the Mangroves, with which the Sides of the Rivers are frequently planted in the Torrid Zone. *Ibid.* p. 74, 75.

Z 4   the

the Windward of the Woods and Marfhes as
poffible ; and if the Anchorage is fafe, one
fhould prefer the open Sea to running up into
Rivers or Creeks (*b*).

Cleannefs and Neatnefs in the Camp is another Article that ought to be particularly regarded. *Pertius, Ramazini,* and moft other
Authors who treat of Camp Difeafes, attribute
thofe of the putrid Kind in a great Meafure to
the Stench and putrid Effluvia arifing from the
Excrements of Men and Beafts, and from the
dead Bodies of Men, Horfes, and other Ani-

(*b*) The higher that Ships fail up the Rivers upon the Coaft
of *Guinea,* the more fickly they become : Such, however, as
keep at Sea beyond the Reach of the Land Breezes (that is, two
or three Leagues at Sea), are for the moft part healthy. *Lind,*
ibid. p. 65. The Malignity of thefe Land Vapours often does
not extend itfelf to any confiderable Diftance, as we know by
manifold Experience. The Troops in *Zealand* were very unhealthy when Admiral *Mitchel's* Squadron, which lay but a little Way from the Shore, enjoyed perfeft Health.— Dr. *Pringle's*
Obfervat. on the Difeafes of the Army, p. 1. chap. vii.—In *July*
and *Auguft* 1744, two Ships, belonging to Admiral *Long's*
Squadron in the *Mediterranean,* lying near the Mouth of the
River *Tyber,* began to be affefted, while others, though at a
very fmall Diftance, but further out at Sea, had not a Man
fick. *Lind, ibid.* p. 66.

mals,

mals, lying unburied in the Neighbourhood of
. Camps, and have in a particular Manner mentioned the Neceffity of burying fuch putrid Subftances.   Dr. *Pringle* has very juftly recommended the Digging of Deep Pits for Privies
in Camp, and covering the Excrements with
Earth daily (*c*) till the Pits are near full, and then
to fill them up with Earth, and dig new ones;
and to punifh every Perfon who fhall eafe himfelf any where in Camp but in the Privies.:
And he remarks, that when the Camp begins
to turn unhealthy, that often the only Means
that will preferve the Health of the Men, is to
change the Ground, and to leave behind all the
Filth and Naftinefs which gave Rife to thofe
putrid Diforders.

In fixed Camps, the ftriking the Tents at

(*c*) The divine Lawgiver *Mofes* has enjoined Cleanlinefs in
the Camp to the *Jews* in a particular Manner, when he fays,
" Thou fhalt have a Place alfo without the Camp, whither
" thou fhalt go forth abroad ; and thou fhalt have a Paddle
" upon thy Weapon, and it fhall be when thou wilt eafe thy-
" felf abroad thou fhalt dig therewith, and fhalt turn back and
" cover that which cometh from thee.   For the Lord thy God
" walketh in the Midft of thy Camp ; therefore fhall thy
" Camp be holy, that he fee no unclean Thing in thee, and
" turn away from thee." *Deuteronomy*, chap. xxiii. verfes 12,
13, 14.

Mid-

Mid-Day in fair Weather, and turning and airing the Straw, and changing it often, as recommended by Dr. *Pringle*, will contribute much to preferve the Health of the Men ; and making the Men wafh themfelves daily, and change their Linen often, and keep themfelves otherwife clean, ought never to be omitted by the Officers.

All military Authors have recommended to Commanders always to have Straw for their Men when they come to their Ground, if poffible ; and to have the Army well fupplied with Provifions; giving proper Encouragement to the Country People, and to Suttlers and Merchants of all Sorts, to bring in every Kind of Provifions and other Neceffaries to Camp; and preventing, as much as poffible, the Soldiers from moroding. And the Commanders of every Corps ought to take Care that their Men form themfelves into Meffes, and that Stoppages be made for buying them Provifions.

In *Germany* every Regiment of the *Britifh* Troops contracted with a Butcher, who was obliged to carry along with them, at all Times, a certain a certain Number of live Sheep and Oxen to kill when wanted, and to fell the Meat at a fixed Price. Every Soldier was obliged to take a certain Quantity, which was paid for by Stoppages made in his Pay; and this Meat was boiled in the Camp Kettles, with fuch Roots and Greens as could be got; by which Means the Men, whenever they could ufe their Kettles, had always a good warm Soop, as well as Meat, to refrefh them after their Fatigues, which, along with their Ammunition Bread, made a good wholefome Food.

In Countries where Fruit is plentiful, a certain Quantity of what is fully ripe, diftributed to the Men in warm Weather, and in hot Climates, will contribute to preferve their Health, though the Abufe of it will prove prejudicial; but unripe and acrid Fruits are always hurtful (*d*).

Water

(*d*) The *Britifh* Soldiers in *Germany* ufed fometimes to hurt their Health by eating great Quantities of raw unripe Apples, Plumbs, and other unripe Fruits; but the foreign Troops had a much better Method of ufing fuch Fruits : They commonly boiled or ftewed them, and eat them with Bread, or with their Meat, which in a great Meafure corrected their bad Qualities.

The

Water is another Article which Commanders endeavour to have their Camp well fupplied with, and therefore they generally encamp near Rivers or Rivulets. Where the
Stream is fmall, Care ought to be taken that its
Courfe be not interrupted, and that no Filth or
Naftinefs, or any Thing that will fpoil or corrupt the Water, be thrown into it.

When there are no Rivers or Rivulets near a
Camp, and the Men are fupplied from Wells,
if the Water is not pure, very often the digging
of deep Pits, and covering the Bottom and Sides
with large Stones, and over thefe a Lay of
Sand, Gravel, or Chalk, will make the Water
pure in a few Hours.

In fixed Camps, where the Water is bad,
Portius (*e*) propofes ftraining it thro' Sand, and
has given Figures of Machines to be ufed for
that Purpofe; but the Method propofed by
Dr. *Lind* is ftill more fimple, which is, to get

The Orders in the *French* Camp, prohibiting the Men from
eating unripe Fruit, were ftrictly complied with every-where in
Germany during the late War.

(*e*) See the Treatife publifhed by Dr. *Luc. Anton. Portius*
in 1686, *de Militis in caftris fanitate tuenda, part.* ii. *cap.* vi.
In this Book we have many ufeful Things mentioned relative
to the Health of Soldiers.

a broad

a broad Cafk with one End ftruck out; then
put a longer Cafk, with both Ends ftruck out,
in the Middle of it; fill the fhort Cafk one-
third with Sand, and the inner longer Cafk
above one-half; fill the Reft of the inner Cafk
with the Water, which will filter through the
Sand, and rife above the Sand in the outer
Cafk, where it may be allowed to run off into
Veffels placed to receive it, by Means of a Cock,
put into the Side of thè outer Cafk, fifteen or
twenty Inches above the Level of the Sand.

Where there are no fuch Conveniences for
purifying the Water, what is ufed for Drink
ought to be mixed with a fmall Proportion of
Spirits, or Wine, or with Vinegar, or Cream of
Tartar, when neither of the other two can
be got; and if the Water be previoufly boiled,
it will be fo much the better.

In Expeditions into warm Countries, where
frefh Water is difficult to be had, a few Stills,
with a proper Apparatus, ought to be carried
out; and after a Landing is made, the Stills
ought to be fet to work for diftilling frefh
Water from Sea Water in the Manner mentioned

tioned by Dr. *Lind* (*e*) ; and although a ſufficient Quantity cannot be diſtilled for ſerving
the whole Army, yet enough may be got in
this Way for the Uſe of the Sick.

When Men are very warm, after long
Marches, and other hard Duties, in Summer;
Officers ſhould endeavour to prevent their
ſwallowing immediately great Quantities of
cold Water, and perſuade them to wait a little
till they cool ; and at ſuch Times, if Spirits
can be got eaſily, to order a ſmall Quantity to
be mixed with the Water in each Man's Can-
teen.

Though the Abuſe of vinous and ſpirituous
Liquors is very deſtructive to the Conſtitution,
yet theſe ſame Liquors, given in Moderation to
Soldiers on Service, during the Times of great
Fatigues, are ſome of the beſt Preſervatives of

(*e*) Dr. *Lind* relates a Number of Experiments of his having
diſtilled Sea Water in different Manners, as recommended by
others ; and concludes, that the beſt Way of getting freſh Water from Salt, is to diſtil the Sea Water by itſelf, without any
Mixture ; and he propoſes having a Still Head to the Coppers
or Iron Pots in which the Meat is dreſſed aboard a Ship. *Ibid.*
nets to p. 84, &c.

Health.

Health. Spirits, for common Ufe, ought to be mixed with Water; and in the hot Climates made into Punch; though in very cold and wet Weather, and in damp Nights, a Glafs of pure Spirits, given to the Men going on Duty, is of great Service; for it is always obferved, that Men are much lefs apt to catch Difeafes from being wet when they are upon a March, or at hard Work, than when they ftand Centinels, or are upon Out-Pofts where they move but little, or when they lie down in their wet Cloaths; and that they are lefs liable to be affected by the Weather after a hearty Meal, or drinking a Glafs of Spirits, or fome generous Liquor, than when their Stomachs are empty.

An Infufion of Bark or other Bitters, and of Garlick, in Spirits, has been found to encreafe their Efficacy as Prefervatives both againft the Effects of Cold and malignant Diftempers. Dr. *Lind* has recommended an Infufion of Garlick in Spirits as one of the beft Stomachics and Diaphoretics he knows in cold wet Weather. And many have recommended a Tincture of the

Bark

Bark (*f*) : Towards, the End of the Year 1743, Mr. *Tough*, one of the Apothecaries to the *Britiſh* military Hoſpital in the late War, then a Mate to a marching Regiment, was ordered to go down the *Rhine* with a Party of Sick, who had the Seeds of the Hoſpital Fever among them, in Bilanders, from *Germany* to *Flanders*. Having had a Caſk or two of Brandy put aboard as Part of the Stores for the Sick, he was afraid left the Men ſhould make too free with the Spirits ; to prevent which he threw in a Quantity of Bark into each Caſk, and gave the Men regularly, Morning and Evening, a Glaſs of this bitter Tincture. At the ſame Time, the Men were kept extremely clean. By theſe Means moſt

(*f*) During the Campaign in *Hungary*, in the Year 1717, Count *Boneval* preſerved both himſelf and Family from Diſorders, by taking himſelf, and making all his Domeſticks take, two or three Times a Day, a ſmall Quantity of Brandy, in which Bark had been infuſed, at a Time when all the Reſt of the Army were infeted with malignant Diſorders. A Regiment in *Italy* continued healthy by the Uſe of the Bark, when the Reſt of the *Auſtrian* Army, who did not purſue the ſame Method, were greatly annoyed with Sickneſs. See *Kramer*. quoted by Dr. *Lind*.

of

of the Sick mended upon the Paffage, without the leaft Appearance of the Malignant Fever again amongft them; whereas, Dr. *Pringle*, who takes Notice of the other Parties who came from the fame Hofpitals in *Germany*, tells us, that the Malignant Fever broke out in a violent Degree, and Half the Number died by the Way, and feveral others foon after their Arrival (*g*).

Commanding Officers ought always to endeavour to proportion the Time the Men are to be upon Duty to the Weather and the Nature of the Climate. The Time of ftanding Centinel in very hard Froft, and in cold wet Weather, or in the Heat of the Day in Summer, when the Weather is very warm, and in hot Climates, ought to be fhorter than when the Weather is dry and more temperate.

The Marches of Troops ought, if poffible, during the Time of very hot Weather, to be made either very early in the Morning, in the Evening, or at Night; and Officers, during the

(*g*) *Obfervat.* part. i. chap. iii.

A a · Courfe

Courfe of an active Campaign, ought to fpare their Men as much as poffible.

And when they are in Quarters, and have nothing to do, they fhould narrowly infpect into their Manner of living; and have them out daily, when the Weather will permit, and exercife them, or march them two or three *Englifh* Miles a-Day, in order to prevent their falling fick for want of Exercife; for Soldiers left to themfelves are very fubject to Difeafes when they come into Quarters after an active Campaign, by leading too indolent a Life, if Officers do not take Care to prevent it. However, at fuch Times, the Exercife ought to be moderate, and the Men fhould not be brought out in wet Weather.

O N

O F

MILITARY HOSPITALS.

WHENEVER Men are feized with Diftempers, they ought immmediately to be feparated from thofe in Health, and either fent to the Regimental (*a*) or General Hofpital.

There is no Part of the Service that requires more to be regarded than the Choice of proper

---

(*a*) Some of the regimental Surgeons in *Germany*, when they took the Field, had always fome fpare Tents carried along with their Medicine Chefts ; and when any of their Men fell fick in Camp, and they could get no Houfe for a regimental Hofpital in Villages, they ordered thefe Tents to be pitched, and had the Ground within well covered with Straw and Blankets, and then put the Sick into them, and there took Care of them till they found an Opportunity of fending them to the Flying Hofpital.

Places for Hofpitals, and the right Management
of them, on which the Health and Strength of
an Army often depends; for in wet unwholefome Seafons, if infectious Diforders get into
the Hofpitals, which poffibly might have been
prevented by proper Care, they often weaken
an Army in a very fhort Time far more than
the Sword of the Enemy.
We have no Account of the particular Manner in which the Antients took Care of their
Sick and Wounded in Times of War; for although we read in *Homer* (*b*) of Surgeons or
Phyficians attending the *Grecian* Camp, and in
Xenophon (*c*) of *Cyrus*'s having appointed Phyficians to his Army; and we learn from *Tacitus* (*d*)
and

(*b*) *Homer* mentions *Podalirius* and *Machaon*, fons of *Æfcula-*
pius, as two excellent Phyficians or Surgeons in the *Grecian*
Army. Vid. *Iliad*, lib. ii. Phyfic and Surgery were antiently
exercifed by the fame Perfons.

(*c*) Vid. *Xenophon. de Inftitut. Cyri*. lib. i. et viii.

(*d*) *Tacitus*, after giving an Account of 50,000 People being
killed by the Fall of an Amphitheatre at *Fidena*, during the
Time of a Shew of Gladiators, has thefe Words : " Ceterum
" poft recentem cladem, patuere procerum domus, fomenta &
" medici paffim præbiti ; fuit urbs per illos dies, quanquam
" mœfta facie veterum inftitutis fimilis, qui magna poft prælia
" faucios '

and *Livy* (*e*), that the wounded *Romans* were received into the Houfes of the Nobility, and had Phyficians to attend them, and were furnifhed with Fomentations and other proper Remedies; and from *Juftin* (*f*), that the *Lacedemonians* followed the fame Method: yet thefe Authors make no Mention of the particular Oeconomy or Manner in which thefe Hofpitals were conducted.

The Hofpitals commonly wanted for an Army acting on the Continent, are,

1. One in the Rear, to follow their Motions, fo as to be always ready to receive the Sick from Camp, which is called the Moveable or Flying Hofpital. 2. One or more, at fome

" faucios largitione & cura fuftentabant." *Vid. lib.* iv. *Annal.* § 63.

(*e*) In *Livy* we find the following Paffage : " Neque immemor ejus quod initio confulatus imbiberat, conciliandi animos plebis, faucios milites curandos dividit patribus. Fabiis plurimi dati, nec alibi majore cura habiti." *Vid. lib.* ii. cap. xlvii.

(*f*) *Juftin* mentions the fame Thing of the *Spartans* after their Defeat at *Sellafia*—" Patentibus omnes domibus faucios " excipiebant, vulnera curabant, lapfos reficiebant." *Vid. lib.* xxviii. cap. iv.

A a 3   Diftance,

Diſtance, in Towns, to receive ſuch of the Sick as can be moved from the Flying Hoſpital, when they are obliged to go from one Place to another ; or when a greater Number of Sick is ſent to them than they can eaſily take Care of (*g*).

Each of the Hoſpitals ought to be provided with Phyſicians, Surgeons Mates, Purveyors, or Commiſſaries, and others, to attend and take Care of the Sick.

Beſides the phyſical People who attend the Hoſpital, one or two Phyſicians ought to go along with the Army to attend the Commander in Chief, and the General and Staff Officers, in Caſe of Sickneſs ; and an Apothecary, provided with a ſmall Cheſt of Medicines, ought to attend at Head Quarters to make up the Preſcriptions of the Phyſicians.

(*g*) When Parties of Sick or Wounded are to be ſent from Camp, or from one Hoſpital to another, Care ought to be taken that they are placed properly in the Waggons ; that they have proper phyſical People, Nurſes, &c. to attend them ; as well as Proviſions, and other Neceſſaries, ſo as to be in no Danger of wanting any Thing while they are on their Journey.

A

A Number of Hofpital Surgeons alfo, with Mates, ought to attend the Army, to be ready in Cafe of an Action. Thefe ought to be attached to the Suite of the Commanders of the different Corps or Brigades, and to be quartered or encamped with them. And each Surgeon fhould be provided with a Waggon or fome Horfes loaded with a proper chirurgical Apparatus, as Inftruments, Bandages, Lint, and other Things neceffary for taking Care of the Wounded.

A fmall Quantity of Medicines, fome Wine, Rice, portable Soop, &c. and Utenfils for a fmall Hofpital, and two, three, or four hundred Sets of Bedding, fhould be carried about with the Army, in Cafe of an Action, for the Ufe of the Wounded, till they have Time to receive Affiftance from the Flying Hofpital. Some of the Bedding ought to be carried on Horfeback, fo as to be at Hand when any of the Surgeons are fent with Detachments that are going upon an Attack.

To prevent crowding the General Hofpitals in Winter Quarters, every Regiment ought to

A a 4   take

take Care of their own Sick, and to have proper Hofpitals fitted up for them.

Dr. *Pringle* has laid down fome very good Directions with regard to the Choice of Places fit for Hofpitals, and the Method of preventing infectious Diforders in them ; and we find many excellent Hints of this Kind in Dr. *Lind* and Monf. *du Hamel*'s Treatifes on the Means of Preferving the Health of Seamen, and fome likewife in Dr. *Brocklefby*'s late Treatife on military Diforders.

In the Time of Service the Commander in Chief generally orders the Hofpitals to be eftablifhed in Towns or Villages that leaft interfere with the military Operations, to which the Sick and Wounded can moft eafily be conveyed ; and which he can beft protect from the Infults of the Enemy (*b*).

In

(*b*) The *Roman* Generals feem to have fent their Sick and Wounded into Towns, in the fame Manner as is done by thofe of the prefent Time. For we read in *Cæfar's Commentaries* of this Method having been practifed on more Occafions than one. In the fixty-fecond Chapter of the third Book, *de Bello Civili*, we have the following Paffage : " Itaque nulla interpofita
fita

In Towns, the Places fitteſt for Hoſpitals are public Buildings, which have large dry airy Apartments, ſituated on a high Ground, where there is a free Draught of Air, and a Command of Water.

In Winter, thcſe Houſes, which have open Fire Places in the Rooms, are always preferable to ſuch as have cloſe Stoves, or no Fire

" ſita mora, ſauciorum modo & ægrorum habita ratione, im-
" pedimenta omnia ſilentio prima nocte ex caſtris *Apolloniam*
" præmiſit, ac conquieſcere ante iter confectum vetuit. His
" una legio miſſa præfidio eſt."—And immediately after, in
chap. lxv. " Itaque præm'ſſis nunciis ad Cn. Domitium Cæſar
" ſcripſit, & quid fieri vellet oſtendit : præſidioque *Apolloniæ*
" cohortibus iv. *Liſſi* i. tres *Orici* relictis; quique erant ex
" vulneribus ægri depoſitis; per Epirum atque Arcarniam iter
" facere cæpit.

And in the twentieth chapter, *de Bello Africano*, we read :
" *Labienus* ſaucios ſuos, quorum numerus maximus fuit, jubet
" in plauſtris deligatos *Adrumentum* deportari."

It would be a right Meaſure, in the Beginning of every War, to ſettle by a Cartel that military Hoſpitals on both Sides ſhould be conſidered as Sanctuaries for the Sick, and mutually protected ; as was agreed upon between the late Earl of *Stairs*, who commanded the *Britiſh* Troops, and the Duke *de Noailles*, who commanded the *French* in the Campaign in *Germany* in the Year 1743. See Dr. *Pringle's Preface.*

Place

Place at all; for an open Fire Place ferves to keep up a free Circulation of Air in a Room, as well as to keep it warm. And for the fame Reafon, where nothing but Stoves can be got to warm the Wards, the Wynd Stoves, which open into the Room or Ward, are vaftly prefer-able to the clofe ones.

Where there are no public Buildings, private Houfes anfwering neareft to the above Defcrip-tion are moft proper for Hofpitals. In gene-ral, Houfes with fmall Rooms make but bad Hofpitals; and very Damp and clofe Places ought by all Means to be avoided.

In Summer, when the Moveable or Flying Hofpital is ordered into Villages, large Barns, and the largeft airy Houfes, are the beft.

Churches, fituated on a dry high Ground, make good Summer Hofpitals; and in Winter, when Neceffity obliged us fometimes to ufe them in *Germany* for this Purpofe, they were found to anfwer very well, when we had Bedfteads or Cradles for the Men to lie upon, and the Wynd Stoves to keep them of a moderate Heat.

In

In making Choice of Houfes for Hofpitals, particular Regard ought to be had to the Privies or Neceffaries; becaufe, where their Smell is offenfive, there is always Danger of infectious Diforders. If, therefore, there be no proper Conveniencies of this Kind about an Hofpital, fuch ought to be contrived fo as to prevent any Danger from their putrid Effluvia. If there be a River near the Hofpital, the Neceffaries may be made above it at a Place where there is a rapid Stream below. In Villages deep Pits may be dug in the Ground behind the Hofpital, and Seats made over them, as in Camp; and a thick Lay of Earth be thrown above the Fœces every Morning, till the Pits are near full, and then they muft be filled up, and others dug to fupply their Place.

When once the Places are fixed upon for Hofpitals, every Ward ought to be made perfectly fweet and clean ; firft, by fcraping and wafhing with Soap and Water, and afterwards with warm Vinegar; and then they ought to be fumigated with the Smoke of wetted Gunpowder and of Aromatics, and afterwards well dried

dried and aired by lighting Fires, and opening the Windows, before any Sick are admitted.

After this the Beds ought to be laid ; in doing of which great Care fhould be taken not to crowd the Wards too much, as nothing corrupts the Air fo much, or fo foon brings on infectious Diforders. Dr. *Pringle* fays, the Beds ought to be laid fo thin, that a Perfon unacquainted with the Danger of bad Air, might imagine there was Room for double or triple the Number. In high lofty Apartments, and in Churches, and other large Places, the Beds may be laid much clofer together than in Rooms with low Cielings. In Churches, or fuch Places, thirty-fix fquare Feet, or a Square of fix Feet by fix, may be allowed for each Man ; but in common Wards we muft allow from forty-two fquare Feet, *i. e.* fix by feven Feet, to fixty-four fquare Feet, or eight by eight, according to the-Height of the Cieling, the Airynefs of the Place, and the Nature of the Difeafes of the Patients.

The Bedding moft fit for Hofpitals, is Palliaffes and Bolfters filled with Straw, Sheets,

and

and Blankets, as they can eafily be wafhed. Feather Beds and Matraffes are apt to retain Infeftion, and cannot be eafily cleanfed. In the fixed Hofpitals, Bedfteads or Cradles may be fet up for laying the Bedding on : But in the Moveable or Flying Hofpital the Bedding muft be, for the moft part, laid on the Floor.

When once the Beds are laid, and the Sick arrive, fome of the Gentlemen belonging to the phyfical Department ought to attend, to diftribute the Sick properly through the Hofpitals.

All the Surgery Patients, fuch as have Wounds, Ulcers, Sores, the Venereal Difeafe, &c. fhould be feparated from the Reft, and put either into particular Wards by themfelves, or into an Hofpital fitted up for that Purpofe under the Direftion of the Surgeons.

Thofe labouring under infeftious Fevers and Fluxes, fhould each of them be placed in good airy Wards by themfelves, where the Beds are laid much thinner than in the other Wards of the Hofpital. If the Flux Wards have a Privy near them, where the Men can eafe themfelves,

felves, without being offenfive either to their own Ward, or any other Part of the Hofpital, they are fo much the fitter for fuch Patients. In the Hofpital I attended at *Bremen*, the Flux Ward had a Neceffary that opened into the River *Wefer*, and at *Natzungen* a deep Pit was dug in the Field about twenty Yards from the Barn where the Flux Men lay, which kept thefe Wards always fweet.

Patients that have got the Itch, or any other infectious Diftemper, ought likewife to be put into feparate Wards by themfelves ; and at all Times a Place fhould be fet apart for thofe who may be taken ill of the Meafles or Small-Pox. A Houfe feparated from the other Hofpitals, with a diftinct Set of Nurfes and other Attendants, bids faireft to prevent the Infection from fpreading.

When once the Sick are properly ranged, the next Care muft be to prevent infectious and malignant Diforders from being generated, and from fpreading amongft the Sick ; which is principally to be effected by keeping the Sick

and

and the Hofpital extremely clean and well-
aired, and the Wards as fweet, and free from
putrid and offenfive Smells, as poffible.

Every fick Man, as foon as he arrives at an
Hofpital, fhould be wafhed with warm Water,
or if there is a warm Bath, or bathing Tub, to
be put intó it; and afterwards be fupplied with
a clean Shirt (*i*) well-aired before he be put to
Bed; and his own dirty Linen fhould be immediately carried to the Wafh-Houfe: And
every Morning each Nurfe ought to carry a
Bucket full of warm Water, and a Piece of
Soap and a Towel, round to each of her
Patients, and make them wafh their Hands
and Face, and their Feet, when dirty.

Every Morning all the Wards ought to be
fcraped and fwept, and afterwards fprinkled
with warm Vinegar; and when dirty, they
ought to be wafhed after the Fires are lighted.

(*i*) Every military Hofpital ought to have a Number of
Shirts belonging to it, for the Ufe of the Sick who arrive without having clean Linen with them. As foon as their own
Shirts are wafhed and dried, or that new ones are provided by
their Regiments, the Hofpital Shirts ought to be taken from
them.

Every

Every Thing in the Wards, and about the Sick, should be kept as clean as possible; the Chamber-Pots and Close-Stools ought to be carried away as soon as used, and immediately emptied and washed before they be brought back.

The Windows of the Wards ought to be kept open to admit fresh Air Morning and Evening, for a longer or shorter Time, according as the Weather will permit.

If the Wards are close, and the Cieling too low, Dr. *Pringle* advises to remove some Part of them, and to open the Garret Story to the Tiles (*k*); and if the Opening of the Windows

(*k*) In Wards which are too close, it has been found that one or two square Holes (of about six or eight, or ten Inches diameter), cut in the Cieling, and a Tube made of Wood fitted to it, and carried up into the Chimney of the Ward above, so as to enter above the Grate, is one of the best Contrivances for procuring a free Circulation of Air ; as the foul Air, which is lightest, and occupies the highest Part of the Ward, finds a free Exit by these Tubes : We have such Tubes now fixed in several of the Wards in *St. George*'s Hospital. A Hole cut above the Door of the Ward, or in the upper Part of the Windows, and one of what are called the *Chamber Ventilators* fixed in it, will answer, where Holes cannot be conveniently cut in the Cieling.

is

is not fufficient to air the Wards, Ventilators of different Kinds, fuch as thofe mentioned by Dr. *Hales* and Dr. *Pringle*, may be ufed, efpecially when the Weather is hot.

In Winter, Fires fhould be lighted in all the Wards where it can be done.

In foreign Countries, when we meet with Hofpitals where there are no Places for open Fires, but only clofe Stoves, different Contrivances may be ufed to renew the Air. Ventilators of different Kinds may be ufed, or Openings made in the Doors and Windows. In Winter 1761-62, fome of the Wards in the Hofpital at *Bremen* which I attended had fuch Stoves. In order to keep up a free Circulation of Air in thofe Wards, I directed large Holes to be cut in the lower Part of the Door in each Ward, and two Grooves to be made on the Outfide of the Door, above and below the Hole, parallel to each other, in which a Board flided ; by means of which, the Hole could be either quite covered or only in Part, or left entirely open ; and I directed a Cafement,

B b   about

about eight or nine Inches fquare, to be made in the upper Corner of each Window. After the Fires were lighted, upon removing the Board which covered the Hole in the Door, and opening the little fquare Windows, a Current of frefh cool Air rufhed into the Ward by the Door, while the heated foul Air found an Exit by the Windows. In very cold Weather, the Opening of the fmall Windows was fufficient ; but in mild Weather, and in Summer, it was necefffary to keep both open.

The Wards fhould be daily fumigated by Means of Aromatics, or wetted Gunpowder thrown on burning Coals, put in an Iron Pot or Chaffern, or with the Steams of warm Vinegar placed in the Middle of the Ward. Dr. *Lind* fays, that although Cleanlinefs and a pure Air contribute much to prevent infectious Diforders, or to check them, yet that they of themfelves are not always fufficient ; but that he feldom or never knew a proper Application of Fire and Smoke to be unfuccefsful in producing the happy Confequence of effectually

purifying

purifying all tainted Places, Materials, and Subftances (*k*).

In all Military Hofpitals, at leaft in the fixed
ónes, one Ward ought to be always kept
empty; and whenever a malignant Fever, or
any other infe\&ious Diforder, breaks out in any
Ward, the Men ought to be removed into this
empty one; and the foul Ward purified, by
wafhing and cleaning it well with Soap and
Water, and then with warm Vinegar ; and afterwards purifying it with Smoke, in the fame
Manner as is practifed in his Majefty's Ships of
War ; and Fires fhould be lighted daily, and
the Windows kept open for fome Time, before any Sick be again admitted into it.

(*k*) Dr. *Lind* tells us, that the Ships of War in his Majefty's
Service are purified by Fire and Smoke, and gives the Procefs
by which it is done; and he fays, that he never heard of any
Ship, which, after being carefully and properly fmoked, did
not immediately become healthy for the Men.—See *Firft Paper on Fevers and Infeation.*—And he obferves, that thefe Steams
and Smoke, which are inoffenfive to the Lungs, befides correcting the bad Quality of the Air, produce another good Effect ; which is, to make both the Patients and Nurfes defirous
of opening the Doors and Windows for the Admiffion of frefh
Air. *Ibid.* p. 51.

As

As foon as any Patient dies, the Body ought to be removed to the Dead Houfe; and the Bedding he lay upon fhould be carried away immediately, and not ufed again till it has been fmoked, well-aired, and wafhed.

All the Linen of Patients in Fevers, Fluxes, and other infectious Diforders, ought to be changed often; and all the foul Linen and foul Bedding of the Hofpital fhould be fmoked with the Fumes of Brimftone, or of wetted Gunpowder, in a Place fet apart for that Purpofe; and Dr. *Lind* advifes to fteep them firft in cold Water, or cold Soap Lees, before putting them in warm Water; as it is dangerous for any Perfon to receive the Steam that may at firft arife, where this Precaution is not ufed.

All the Cloaths, of Soldiers who die in Hofpitals, ought to be fent to the Smoke Houfe, and be well fumigated, and afterwards aired, before they are put up in the Store-Houfe.

The next Thing to be confidered about a Military Hofpital is the Diet of the Patients, which fhould confift of good wholefome Provifions,

vifions, that can be purchafed eafily, and at a cheap Rate (*k*).

Good Bread (*l*) is a ftanding Article of Provifions for an Hofpital in all Countries and in all Climates; and a certain Quantity of it ought to be diftributed to each Man daily.

The Breakfaft and Supper in moft Military Hofpitals muft be made of Water Gruel or Rice Gruel; as either Rice or Oatmeal can be got in moft Places, and are very portable.— Water Gruel is in general preferable to the Rice Gruel, becaufe moft Patients naufeate the Rice Gruel, after eating it for fome Days, but not the Water Gruel, as every Perfon, who has attended the Military Hofpitals, muft have ex-

(*k*) The *French*, and many other Nations, give their Patients Meat Soops in acute Difeafes, and after capital Operations; and they allow them but li tle Bread or other Preparations of Vegetable Subftances: But thefe Meat Soops without Bread do not nourifh the Patient fufficiently, and tend too much to the Putrefcent; and this is one Reafon why more Sick die in the *French* than in the *Britifh* Hofpitals.

(*l*) On Expeditions where a Siege is expected, a Quantity of Flour ought to be carried cut, and a Number of portable Ovens for baking bread for the Sick, which may be put up after the Troops have made good their Landing.

B b 3   perienced.

perienced. Where both Rice and Oatmeal can be had, Rice Gruel may be ufed two or three Times a Week by Way of Variety.

But although Rice Gruel is not fo proper for conftant Ufe, yet Rice fhould always make an Article among the Stores for an Hofpital, as it is ufeful for making Rice Water for Drink ; and it can be boiled or ground, and made into a light Pudding, and in fhort may be ufed in a Variety of Forms to make a good and wholefome Food for the Sick.

Oatmeal is cheaper than Rice, and can be procured almoft every-where in *Europe*, where Armies make Campaigns ; as Oats make fuch a great Article in the Forage for Horfes. And a fufficient Quantity can at any Time be ground into Meal for the Ufe of the Sick, at the Mills which are employed for making Flour for the Bakery, if there be none nearer the Hofpital.

In Countries where neither Oatmeal nor Rice can be had, *Indian* or fome other Corn, which is known to be wholefome, and which the Country affords, may be employed in their Place.

When

When freſh Meat can be got, the Men who are on full Diet, and the Nurſes and other Servants about the Hoſpital, ſhould have Meat for Dinner; and the Meat that is boiled for them ought to make Broth for the Sick who are kept on a low or middle Diet. Some Barley or Rice ſhould be added to the Broth; and a ſmall Quantity of Carrots, Turnips, or other Vegetables, boiled along with them, will make it more agreeable to the Taſte.

On Expeditions where nothing but ſalted Meat can be had, a Quantity of portable Soop ſhould always be carried out for the Uſe of the Sick; which with Water and ſome Barley, and freſh Vegetables, when they can be got, will make a good Soop or Broth. On ſuch Occaſions, the Dinner ought to conſiſt of Soop and Bread, or of light Puddings made of Flour or of Rice, of boiled Rice or Barley, or of Panado, &c.

Nurſes and recovered Men may be allowed ſalted Meat twice or thrice a Week.

The common Drink of Military Hoſpitals ought to be Rice and Barley Water, with a

ſmall

fmall Proportion of Spirits and Sugar. Small Beer is a good Drink where it can be eafily procured; as is Wine and Water, or a very fmall Negus, or very weak Punch in warm Climates.

Befides this Diet, extraordinary Indulgences may be occafionally allowed to particular Patients, as Wine, Brandy, Sugar, Milk. And the Phyficians and Surgeons ought to have a difcretionary Power to order a Vegetable or any other proper Diet for Patients in the Scurvy, or any other particular Complaints.

The

The Eftablifhed Diet of a Military Hofpital may be,

	Breakfaft.	*Dinner.*	*Supper.*
Full Diet,	One Pint of Water or Rice Gruel. Water Gruel made with 3 or 4 Ounces of Oatmeal, a little common Salt, and with or without a little Sweet Oil, and two Spoonfuls of Wine. Rice Gruel made with two Ounces of Rice, one Spoonful of fine Flour, a little common Salt and Sugar.	One Pound of boiled frefh Meat.	As Breakfaft.
Middle Diet,	Ditto.	One Pint of Broth, half Pound of boiled Meat.	Ditto.
Low Diet,	Ditto, or according to the Patient's Appetite.	One Pint of Broth, or half a Pint of Panado, with two Spoonfulls of Wine, and a Quarter of an Ounce of Sugar.	Ditto.

The daily Allowance of Bread to be one Pound to each Man.

The

The common Drink for thofe on full and middle Diet to be Rice or Barley Water, with two Spoonfuls of Brandy to each Pint, and a Quarter of an Ounce of Lump Sugar; fmall Beer, or very weak Punch; or Wine and Water, two Ounces of Wine to a Pint of Water, and a Quarter of an Ounce of Sugar. The Quantity not to exceed three Pints *per* Day.

Thofe on low Diet to have Rice or Barley Water as above, with or without Wine or Brandy.

The Diet Boards hung up in the Hofpitals may be made with the following Columns, nearly as they were with us in *Germany*.

Regiments.	Mens Names.	Diet. F. M. L.	Wine, ½ Pints.	Brandy. Ounces.	Milk. ¼ Pints.	Sugar. Ounces.

When

When fuch Diet Boards are kept in an Hof-pital, and the Mens Names and Regiments are once wrote down, the Patients may with very little Trouble be put upon the full, middle, or low Diet, with fo much of the above-mentioned Extraordinaries as may be judged proper.

If any Thing elfe be wanted for the Sick, the Phyfician ought to give a particular Order in Writing for it, the Columns here marked being only for fuch Things as are moft fre-quently wanted.

It fhould be a general Rule in all Military Hofpitals, that, when a Party of Sick arrives, every Man may have immediately a Mefs of Water Gruel given him, and afterwards be put on low Diet till it is ordered otherwife by the Phyfician or Surgeon who attends him.

It is not to be fuppofed that the Diet here mentioned can be ftrictly kept to in all Parts of the World; for it muft often be varied accor-ding to the Difference of the Climates, and to the Provifion of the Countries where the Scene of War may be.

Whenever

Whenever a Moveable or Flying Hofpital is
to attend an Army, a Quantity of Bedding, and
of all Utenfils for forming an Hofpital, ought
to be put up in the Waggons, together with
Provifions of different Kinds, fuch as Oatmeal,
Rice, Sago, Brandy, Wine, Sugar, &c. A Butcher with a Stock of live Cattle, and a Baker
with a proper Quantity of Flour for making
Bread ought conftantly to attend ; and a Number of empty Waggons fhould likewife be always in Readinefs, to tranfport the Sick when
the Hofpital moves, or when a Party is to be
fent to the fixed Hofpitals.

When Troops go upon an Expedition, befides the common Hofpital Ships, another Ship
ought to be properly fitted up for the Reception of fick Officers (*m*) ; and every Hofpital
Ship ought to be fupplied with all Sorts of

(*m*) If there be no Ship fitted up for the Reception of fick
Officers, thofe who are taken ill on Expeditions muft be in a
moft miferable Situation ; as there is no Place to receive them
in the common Hofpital Ships, they muft remain almoft without Affiftance in a crowded Cabin amongft People in Health ; as
was the Cafe in fome of our Expeditions during the late War.

Pro-

Provifions, and other Neceffaries fit for forming an Hofpital, before they leave *England*.—
And one or more armed Veffels loaded with
Provifions, Wine, and all Sorts of Neceffaries
for the Sick, ought to attend them ; or if the
Expedition be intended for the warm Climates,
thefe Veffels ought to go before the Fleet to
take up Wine and Fruits, fuch as Lemons,
Oranges, &c. Vegetables of different Kinds,
and a live Stock for the Ufe of the Sick.

All Hofpitals attending Expeditions fhould
carry out among their Stores a Number of
large Tents for lodging the Sick and Wounded
immediately on making good their Landing.
Where a Siege is expected which will take up
Time, and where no Accommodations for the
Sick can be had till the Siege is over, a Ship or
two, with Boards, and other Neceffaries for
building large Sheds, or temporary Hutts, for
the Sick, as propofed by Dr. *Brocklefby*, ought
to go along with the Fleet, or meet them at
the Place of their Deftination. Such thatched
Sheds, or Hutts, are very neceffary in the warm
Climates, as the perpendicular Rays of the Sun,

beating

beating upon Canvafs, make Tents intolerably hot. When any of our own Settlements
happen to be near the Place attacked, a fixed
Hofpital may be eftablifhed there; either in
Houfes, if proper ones can be found; or in
temporary Sheds or Hutts erected for that Purpofe; and fome Veffels, properly fitted up,
may be kept going with the Sick and Wounded, and bringing back the recovered Men.

At every Military Hofpital a Serjeant's Guard
ought to mount; and Centinels be placed at
the Doors of the Hofpital, 1. To prevent all
Vifitors, who have not proper Leave, from
coming into the Hofpitals; as fuch People oftentimes crowd the Wards, difturb the Sick,
and are apt to catch infectious Diftempers, and
to fpread them among the Troops. 2. To
take Care the Patients do not go out of the
Hofpital without having a Ticket (*n*) of Leave
for that Purpofe, figned by the Phyfician, Sur-

(*n*) At every Hofpital there ought to be a Number of printed
Tickets lying ready to be filled up and figned by the Phyficians
and Surgeons, and no Man ought to be allowed to go out
without a Ticket fo figned.

geon,

geon, or Apothecary, belonging to the Hofpital. 3. To prevent fpirituous Liquors, or other Things of that Kind, being clandeftinely carried into the Hofpital.

The Serjeant of the Guard, attended by the Ward Mafter, ought, every Morning, to go round the Wards to call a Roll, and fee that every Man is in his Ward ; and to do the fame at Night before the Hofpital Doors are fhut, and at this Time to order every Perfon out of the Hofpital who does not belong to it. And the Serjeant, every Morning, ought to report to the Phyfician, Surgeon, or Apothecary, . every Man's Name who was found to be abfent at Roll-calling ; and whether he found every Thing regular and in good Order in going his Rounds.

Every large Military Hofpital ought to have one Head Nurfe, and a fufficient Number of other Nurfes, to attend and take Care of the Sick.

Orders to the following Purport, hung up in every Military Hofpital, would ferve to fhew the Nurfes and Patients what their Duty is, and

and to maintain Regularity and good Order through the whole Hofpital.

Matron, or Head Nurſe.

Every Matron, or Head Nurſe, is to go round all the Wards of the Hofpital at leaſt twice a Day, Morning and Evening; to ſee that the Nurſes keep their Wards clean; that they behave themſelves ſoberly and regularly, and give due Attendance to their Patients; and to examine the Diet of the Patients, and ſee that it is good and well dreſſed; and if ſhe finds any Thing amiſs, to report the ſame to the Phyſician, Surgeon, or Apothecary, of the Hofpital.

Common Nurſes.

1. The Nurſes are to give due Attendance to their Patients; and to keep them always as neat and clean, as the Nature of their Diſtempers will admit of; to give them their Diet regularly; to be particularly careful to ſee them take the Medicines ordered by the Phyſicians,

according

according to the Directions given; to report to the Phyfician, Surgeon, or Apothecary, any Faults or Irregularities which any of their Patients may have committed; and to acquaint the Ward Mafter and Head Nurfe of the Death of any of their Patients as foon as it happens, that proper Care may be taken of their Cloaths and Effects.

2. They are to keep their Wards extremely clean, to fprinkle them every Morning with Vinegar, and to fumigate them with the Smoke of wetted Gunpowder, or of Frankincenfe, or any other Aromatics that may be thought proper; in fair Weather to keep open the Windows of their Wards, twice or thrice a Day, for a longer or fhorter Time, as the Weather will permit; to attend at the Steward's Room for the Provifions of the Patients at the Hours appointed for that Purpofe; and to pay implicit Obedience to the Matron, or Head Nurfe, in what relates to their Duty; and punctually to obey all Orders they receive from the Phyfician, Surgeon, or Apothecary, of the Hofpital.

C c　　　　　　3. They

3. They are to keep themſelves clean and decently dreſſed, and to obſerve the ſtricteſt Rules of Sobriety; remembering, that if any one is found intoxicated with Liquor, that ſhe is immediately to be ſent to the Guard, and afterwards diſcharged.

4. They are not to abſent themſelves from their Wards, unleſs when employed in the Diſcharge of their Duty; nor to go out of the Hoſpital to which they belong, without having a Ticket of Leave ſigned by the Phyſician, Surgeon, Apothecary, or Head Nurſe, belonging to the Hoſpital.

5. They are not to throw Naſtineſs of any Kind out at the Windows, but to carry it to the common Neceſſaries, and to empty the Chamber Pots and Cloſe-ſtools as ſoon as uſed, and be careful to waſh them before they bring them back.

6. They are not, upon any Pretence whatever, to alter the Diet ordered by the Phyſicians or Surgeons to the Patients on the Diet Boards; nor to ſuffer their Patients to uſe any other Diet than what is allowed by the Hoſpital;

2   nor

nor are they to bring, or allow others to bring, Meat, fpirituous Liquors, or other Things of that Kind, into their Wards, except what is allowed by the Phyficians or Surgeons. Whenever any Thing of this Kind is found in any of the Wards, it ought immediately to be thrown into the common Neceffary; and if it be found in the Cuftody of a Nurfe, fhe ought to be confined in the Guard, or difcharged.

7. Nurfes guilty of great Neglect of Duty, or of getting drunk and ufing their Patients ill, or of ftealing, or concealing or taking away the Effects of Men who die in the Hofpital, are to be immediately fent to the Guard, and reported to the Commanding Officer of the Place, that they may be tried by a Court-Martial, and be confined, whipped, or otherwife punifhed, as the military Law directs; all Followers of Armies on foreign Service being equally fubject to the military Law as the Soldiers themfelves.

Patients.

1. All fick Soldiers, on their Arrival at a Military Hofpital, are to be wafhed all over with

warm

warm Water, or to go into a warm Bath;
and afterwards to waſh their Face and
Hands every Morning, and their Feet occaſionally, with warm Water and Soap, brought
round every Morning by the Nurſes for that
Purpoſe; and they ought to comb their Head
every Day. If they be too weak to waſh and
comb themſelves, it is to be done by their
Nurſes.

2. Every Patient is to be ſhaved and have
clean Linen twice a Week, or oftener if requi-
ſite.

3. They are punctually to obey the Directions given them, and to take the Medicines ordered by the Phyſician; and none to be allowed to go out of the Hoſpital without a Ticket
of Leave ſigned by the Phyſician, Surgeon, or
Apothecary, of the Hoſpital.

4. They muſt commit no Diſorder or Riot,
but in all Reſpects behave themſelves well.

5. If any Man diſobeys the Orders he receives from the Phyſicians or Surgeons, or is
irregular in Conduct, gets drunk, and com-
mits Riots in the Hoſpital, or is found guilty
of

of Theft or other Crimes, the fame is to be reported to the Commanding Officer of the Place, and he to be tried by a Court-Martial, and punifhed as foon as his Strength will permit.

In conducting the Military Hofpitals, we found that it was always right to difcharge the Patients from the fick Hofpitals as foon as they were recovered, and to fend them either to Billet, or to a convalefcent Hofpital ; becaufe recovered Men are always the moft riotous ; befides they crowded the Hofpitals, and were in Danger of catching frefh Diforders from thofe who were fick ; and therefore the recovering Men in every Hofpital ought to be reviewed once or twice a Week by the Phyfician or Surgeon, and the Names of fuch Men as are well enough, to be marked; in order that they may be fent the next Day to the convalefcent Hofpital, or to Billet. A Return of thofe marked for Billet ought immediately to be fent to the Officers on convalefcent Duty.

When a convalefcent Hofpital is eftablifhed, it ought to be put under proper Regula-

C c 3   tions ;

tions; the following are thofe which I drew up for that eſtabliſhed at *Oſnabruck* in *April* 1761, and which were found to anſwer the Purpoſe intended.

Regulations for a Convaleſcent Hoſpital.

1. That this Hoſpital be entirely occupied by ſuch Men as are recovered from Diſeaſes; that no Men be ſent there but thofe whofe Names are returned to the Purveyor's Office by the Phyſician or Surgeon of the Hoſpital.

2. That all the Patients ſhall be upon full Diet, unlefs in particular Cafes it be ordered otherwife by the Phyſician or Surgeon.

3. That all the Patients ſhall breakfaſt, dine, and ſup, at regular ſtated Hours, in the Hall appointed for that Purpofe: Breakfaſt to be ready at nine, Dinner at one, and Supper at ſeven o'Clock in the Evening.

4. That no Patient ſhall carry up any Victuals into the Wards appointed for ſleeping in; and if any Patient does not attend at the regular Hours of Meals, no Allowance of Victuals ſhall

shall be made him in the Place of such Meals, unlefs he has been abfent on Hofpital Bufinefs, or been confined to Bed by Sicknefs.

5. That as foon as the Men are come down Stairs to Breakfaft, the Wards in which they fleep fhall be cleaned out and fprinkled with Vinegar, and the Windows opened to air them.

6. That the Doors of this Hofpital fhall be locked every Night at eight o'Clock, and no Man be allowed to come in or go out after that Time. The Doors to be opened again at feven 'Clock in the Morning.

7. That the faid Hofpital is to be vifited two or three Times a Week by the Phyfician, Surgeon, and Apothecary, who are to fee that the above Orders are complied with; to examine the Diet, and take Care that every Thing is carried on properly ; and to prefcribe for any little Diforders the Men may be affected with.

8. That one of the Hofpital Mates be appointed to vifit this Hofpital daily, to adminifter any Medicines which may have been pre-

fcribed by the Phyfician; to apply any Dreffings ordered by the Surgeon; and to acquaint
the Phyfician or Surgeon if any of the Men be
fo bad as to require their Attendance, or to be
fent back again to the Sick Hofpital.

9. That for the better executing thefe Regulations, orderly Serjeants or Corporals be appointed for the Care of the Men; who fhall
mount a Guard of fix or more of fuch of the
Patients of the faid Hofpital as are fit for this
Duty—That the Serjeants are to call a Roll of
all the Patients regularly three Times a Day,
before Breakfaft, Dinner, and Supper; to fee
that the Men behave themfelves foberly and
decently; and that they keep themfelves clean,
and commit no Riots; and to confine in the
Guard fuch as commit Riots and other Irregularities, or whom they find drunk, or who ftay
out all Night; and to report the fame to the
Officer on Duty.

10. That an Officer on convalefcent Duty do
vifit the faid Hofpital daily at the Times of
Roll-calling, to fee that every Thing be carried
on properly; and to receive the Reports from
the

the Serjeants, and give what Orders he may think proper for the better regulating the faid Hofpital.

11. That if at any Time it fhould happen that there are more Convalefcents than the Hofpital can hold conveniently, a Revew be made of all the Patients, and the ftrongeft and moft healthy be fent to Billet.

12. That a Review be always made, when any Party is going to join the Army, to pick out the Men who are fit to join their Regiments.

The Phyfical Officers employed in the Military Hofpitals, are Phyficians, Surgeons, and Apothecaries.

No Perfon ought to be appointed a Phyfician to the Army, or Military Hofpitals, without previoufly undergoing the fame Examination at the College of Phyficians, as thofe do who enter Fellows and Licentiates of the College, that none but proper Perfons may be employed. On fuch Examinations the Phyfician General to the Army ought to be allowed to fit as one of the Cenfors of the College.

The

The Surgeons are all obliged to pass an Examination at Surgeons Hall before they are appointed, and the Apothecaries ought in like Manner to pass an Examination at Apothecaries Hall.

The Mates employed in the Service ought, previous to their Appointment, to be examined both in Surgery and Pharmacy, as the Service commonly requires their acting in both Branches.

The Direction of all Military Hospitals ought always to be committed to the Physicians, who have the immediate Care of Hospitals.

When an Army is acting on a Continent, and there is a Number of Hospitals in different Places, the Physician who attends the Commander in Chief ought to be made Physician General and Director of the Hospitals, with proper Appointments.; and all Orders from Head Quarters ought to go immediately thro' this Channel.

Every other Physician at the different Hospitals ought to direct every Thing about the

Hospital

Hofpital which he attends, and his Orders ought to be punctually obeyed ; and he ought to keep up a conftant Correfpondence with the Phyfician General ; acquainting him from Time to Time with the State of the Hofpital, and what is wanted for it ; and he ought punctually to obey whatever Orders he receives from the Phyfician General.

If there be feparate Hofpitals for the Surgery Patients, the eldeft Surgeon ought to direct every Thing in the Hofpital he attends; and when any Thing is wanted for his Hofpital, to report the fame to the Phyfician General.

The directing and purveying Branches ought never to be entrufted to the fame Perfon, as the Temptation of accumulating Wealth has at all Times, and in all Services, given Rife to the grofleft Abufes, which have been a great Detriment to the Service, as well as to the poor wounded and fick Soldiers, and has occafioned the Lofs of many Lives. And therefore neither the Phyfician General, nor any of the Phyficians or Surgeons of the Army, or any other Perfon concerned in the Direction of the Military

tary

tary Hofpitals, ought ever to act as Purveyor or Commiffary ; nor ought they ever to have any Thing to do with the Accounts, Contracts, or any other Money Affairs relating to the Hofpital ; and if ever they be found to intermeddle in thefe Affairs, they ought to be immediately difmiffed the Service.

The purveying or commiffariate Branch ought to be entirely diftinct from the phyfical. The Purveyors or Commiffaries ought punctually to obey whatever Orders they receive from the Phyficians or Surgeons ; to provide every Thing for the Hofpital ; to keep regular Accounts of all the Men who come into, or go out of the Hofpitals ; and from Time to Time to make Returns to Head Quarters of all the Men in Hofpitals ; and their Accounts ought to be controuled by fuch Perfons as the Government may think proper.

Every Phyfician and Surgeon of a Military Hofpital ought to vifit the Sick at regular ftated Hours, and the Mates to attend and go round with them, and receive and execute their Orders.

Every

Every Mate ought to have a certain Number of Patients allotted him, for whom he is to make up all Medicines, drefs all Sores, and execute whatever Orders he receives from the Phyfician, Surgeon, or Apothecary. That the Mates may know and execute their Duty, proper Orders in Writing fhould be hung up in the Apothecaries Shop for that Purpofe. The following are thofe which I gave out at all the Hofpitals I attended in *Germany*.

Orders for the Mates.

1. That all the Gentlemen do attend at the Apothecaries Shop every Morning at eight o'Clock, to affift in making up the common Medicines of the Day, and afterwards to go round the Hofpitals with the Phyficians and Surgeons.

2. That every Mate have a Book for writing the Prefcriptions of the Phyficians in, which is to be kept in the following Order.— Firft, to mark the Patient's Name and Regiment; then the Day of his Entry into the Hof-

pital

pital and his Diforder ; then the Prefcriptions of the Phyfician ; and after all the Day of his Difcharge, or of his Death. *Ex. gr.*

John Clarke, 20th Regiment. *Jan.* 1. Fever.

Jan. 1. V. S. unc. x.—H. falin. cum pulv. contrayerv. 4ʳ. die.—2. Emplaft. veficat. dorfo, &c.

Difcharged or dead *Jan.* 28.

3. That every Mate make up himfelf the Phyfician's Prefcriptions for his own Patients, and afterwards go round and adminifter them, or give them to his Patients with proper Directions ; that he bleed his own Patients, and drefs any flight Sores they may have, which do not require their being fent to the Surgery Hofpital.

4. That every Mate go round amongft his Patients in the Evening, to fee that every Thing is well conducted, and to report to the Phyfician or Apothecary if any Thing extraordinary happens.

5. That

5. That two of the Mates attend all Day at the Apothecary's Shop to receive any Sick that may arrive, and to place them properly; to make up what Medicines they may immediately want; to order each of them a Mefs of Water Gruel; and if any Thing extraordinary occurs, to fend an orderly Man to acquaint the Phyfician or Apothecary with the fame. The orderly Mates to make up likewife for Officers, or others, all Prefcriptions fent to the Apothecary's Shop through the Day.

A Joint of Meat, roafted or boiled, for Dinner, and a Bottle of Wine, was allowed to the orderly Mates, by Lord *Granby*'s Order, that they might not abfent themfelves from their Duty.—Where there was Conveniency for it, a Mate lodged in the Hofpital.

The Apothecary ought to take Care of the Medicines; to go round the Hofpitals in the Morning before the Time of the Phyfician's vifiting; to fee that the Wards are in proper Order; that the Nurfes and other Servants have done their Duty; to examine into the State of the Sick, and to fee that the Provifions

are

are good; and make a faithful Report of all
thefe Things to the Phyfician when he arrives.
—To take Care that the Mates prepare in the
Morning the Medicines that are commonly
wanted for the Day ; and that they afterwards
make up faithfully the Prefcriptions of the
Phyfician ; to go round the Hofpital again in
the Evening, to fee that the Sick have got their
Medicines regularly; and to make the fame
Enquiries as in the Morning.

The Apothecary fhould always be lodged
near the Hofpital, to affift in Cafe of any Accidents happening, or of Sick arriving at the
Hofpital.

When there are any ftrong infectious Diforders in Military Hofpitals, the phyfical Gentlemen may ufe the following Precautions to guard
themfelves againft Infection.

1. Never to vifit the Sick with an empty
Stomach ; but to eat Breakfaft before they go
into the Hofpital.

2. To have a Suit of Cloaths referved for
vifiting the Hofpital, and a waxed Linen Coat
to wear above them in going round the Wards ;
and

and as foon as they have come out of the Hofpital, to wafh and change their Linen and
Cloaths.

3. Before they go into the Wards, to order
that they be well cleaned out, and fprinkled
with Vinegar, and afterwards fumigated, and
aired by opening the Windows, or by working
the Ventilators.

4. If the Infection be very ftrong, to take a
Glafs of the fpirituous Tincture of the Bark
juft before they go into the Hofpital.

5. To put fmall Rolls of Lint, dipped in
camphorated Spirits, up the Noftrils, and to
direct a Veffel, with warm camphorated Vinegar, to be carried round, and held near the
Patients they are examining.

6. In examining Patients affected with the
Petechial Fever, or any other malignant Diftempers, to ftand at fome little Diftance, and
afk what Queftions they may think proper;
and when they come near, to feel the Pulfe,
and examine the Skin, not to infpire while
their Head is near the Patient's Body; but
after being fully fatisfied in thefe Points, to re-

D d   tire

tire a little, and aſk what other Queſtions may be neceſſary.

It would be right to eſtabliſh ſome military Rank for every commiſſioned Officer of the Hoſpital on Service, and to ſettle the ſame Subordination in the phyſical as in the military Department. By theſe Means, the Service would be carried on with greater Order, and more Advantage to the Sick.

And it would be right, in Times of War, to add a Clauſe in the Mutiny Bill to allow any military Officer on convaleſcent Duty to call in the commiſſioned phyſical Officers to aſſiſt in making up a Court-Martial, when there are not a ſufficient Number of military Officers in a Place, to try convaleſcent Soldiers guilty of Crimes. For in Times of Service, very often a ſufficient Number of military Officers cannot be ſpared to be on Duty at the different Military Hoſpitals ; and at all ſuch Places the Convaleſcents are generally very diſorderly, when they know that there is not a ſufficient Number of Officers to form a Court-Martial for puniſhing them. Where-

ever

ever there are a fufficient Number of military Officers, no phyfical Officer ought ever to be called upon as a Member of a Court-Martial.

Men, in Time of Service, are often apt to faunter in and about Hofpitals, and there learn all Manner of Debaucheries, and lofe all Senfe of Difcipline; and therefore, to keep up Order and Decorum, there ought to be, at every Fixed and every large Military Hofpital, a military Infpector or Commander, an Officer of known Activity and Probity; and a Number of Officers on convalefcent Duty fufficient to form a Court-Martial whenever required.

The Duty of the Military Infpector, or Commander, fhould be, to take Care of all Convalefcents on Billet; to fee that the Officers under him do their Duty, and maintain the fame Regularity and Difcipline among the Men belonging to their refpective Corps, as if they were with their Regiments; and that the Men attend the Parade and Roll-calling; and that they always appear neat and clean.

He ought, from Time to Time, to vifit the Hofpitals; to fee if they are kept clean; to

enquire

enquire if the Men behave well, if the Diet is good, and the Officers, Nurfes, and Servants, do their Duty; and if he finds any Thing amifs, to report the fame to the Phyficians and Surgeons of the Hofpital, or to the Purveyor or Commiffary, or others, under whofe Department it may be, that the fame may be immediately rectified; and if he finds that the fuperior Officers of the Hofpital overlook fuch Abufes, notwithftanding his Reprefentations, to report the fame immediately to the Head Quarters.

He ought to order one of the Officers on convalefcent Duty to vifit the Hofpitals daily, to make the Enquiries above-mentioned, and to give him a Report of the fame in Writing.

The Purveyor or Commiffary ought to make a Return to him twice or thrice a Week of every Man admitted into, or difcharged from, the Hofpitals, or who dies in them; marking in the Return the Name of every Man, and the Company and Regiment he belongs to; that he may report the fame to the Officers of the different Brigades or Regiments.

The

The Military Infpector ought to have the Power of providing Billets for all Officers and Soldiers about Hofpitals; and the Names of all Men to be difcharged from Hofpitals fhould be fent to him the Day before they are dif- charged, that he may provide Billets for them; and next Day the Men ought to march from the Hofpitals to the Parade, to receive their Billets, and the Orders of the Military Infpector, and of the Officers of the Corps they belong to.

The Military Infpector ought to fee that the Arms of the fick Men, and the Arms and Cloaths of thofe who die and are lodged in the Magazines, be properly taken Care of; and that the Stores of the different Regiments be properly looked after.

As the Service often makes it neceffary at Military Hofpitals, where the Number of Sick is great, to employ the convalefcent Soldiers (*l*)

(*l*) In the *French* Hofpitals there are always a Number of Men who attend their Sick who belong to the Hofpital, fo that they have no Occafion to employ their Convalefcents, as we are often obliged to do, where the Sick are attended by Nurfes, who are commonly Soldiers Wives, and not fo capable of doing fuch laborious Work as the Men.

as

as orderly Men and Servants about Hoſpitals, all Men thus employed ought to have a ſpecial Leave from the Military Inſpector for ſo doing ; and no Man ſhould be employed in any Capacity as a Servant about an Hoſpital, who at that Time is on the Books as a Patient. And all Men employed about the Hoſpital ought to be reviewed once a Week by the Military Inſpector, and likewiſe whenever a Party of Convaleſcents is going to join the Army, or their Regiments ; that no Man may be allowed to remain with the Hoſpital, after he is fit to do Duty in his Regiment.

When the Military Inſpector is abſent, the eldeſt Officer on convaleſcent Duty ought to act in his Place.

Every Officer ſent on convaleſcent Duty ought, as ſoon as he arrives at the Place where the Hoſpital is, to wait on the Commandant, or Military Inſpector ; to acquaint him of his Arrival, and to receive his Commands. He ought then to go to the Purveyor or Commiſ-ſary's Office, to get a Liſt of all the Soldiers who are in or about the Hoſpital, and belong to the

the Regiment or Brigade he is employed for, wherein thofe on Billet are diftinguifhed from thofe in Hofpitals. The next Day he ought to parade all thofe marked on Billet, to fee if the Number of Men agrees with the Lift given him, and to examine in what State each Man is, and how he is employed; and then he ought to go round the Hofpitals, attended by an orderly Serjeant, to fee all the Men in the Hofpitals, and to know if the Lift given him at the Purveyor's Office was right; and afterwards he ought to fend every Day a Serjeant or Corporal to fee the Men in Hofpitals, and to report to him when any Men are difcharged or die.—And he ought to procure from the Military Infpector a Return of all the Men of his Corps, who are either admitted into, or difcharged from Hofpitals, on the Days when fuch Returns are made. He ought to make all his Men on Billet appear regularly on the Parade at Roll-calling, and to oblige them to keep themfelves clean and their Arms in good Order, and to endeavour to preferve the fame Regularity and Difcipline as when they are

with

with their Regiments. And whenever a Party is to be fent to join their Regiments, he ought to have all his Men particularly examined; and thofe Men who are found to be perfectly recovered, fhould be fent to their Regiments.

If every Officer on convalefcent Duty conform to thefe Directions, no Man can ever be detained without his Knowledge in or about Hofpitals, as he muft always know where every Man is, in what State of Health, and how he is employed; and may at any Time be able to make a Return to the Brigade or Regiment for which he is employed, of every Man who is admitted, difcharged, or dies in the Hofpital.

F   I   N   I   S.

www.ingramcontent.com/pod-product-compliance
Lightning Source LLC
Chambersburg PA
CBHW032307280326

41932CB00009B/733